Endoscopic Closure Techniques: Endoscopic Clipping over the Scope (C-OTS) and Endoscopic Suturing

Editors

ROY SOETIKNO
TONYA KALTENBACH

GASTROINTESTINAL ENDOSCOPY
CLINICS OF NORTH AMERICA

www.giendo.theclinics.com

Consulting Editor
CHARLES J. LIGHTDALE

January 2020 • Volume 30 • Number 1

ELSEVIER

1600 John F. Kennedy Boulevard • Suite 1800 • Philadelphia, Pennsylvania, 19103-2899

http://www.theclinics.com

**GASTROINTESTINAL ENDOSCOPY CLINICS OF NORTH AMERICA Volume 30, Number 1
January 2020 ISSN 1052-5157, ISBN-13: 978-0-323-75421-7**

Editor: Kerry Holland
Developmental Editor: Donald Mumford

Gastrointestinal Endoscopy Clinics of North America (ISSN 1052-5157) is published quarterly by Elsevier Inc., 360 Park Avenue South, New York, NY 10010-1710. Months of issue are January, April, July, and October. Business and Editorial Offices: 1600 John F. Kennedy Blvd., Suite 1800, Philadelphia, PA, 19103-2899. Periodicals postage paid at New York, NY and additional mailing offices. Subscription prices are $359.00 per year for US individuals, $655.00 per year for US institutions, $100.00 per year for US and Canadian students/residents, $399.00 per year for Canadian individuals, $774.00 per year for Canadian institutions, $476.00 per year for international individuals, $774.00 per year for international institutions, and $245.00 per year for international students/residents. To receive student/resident rate, orders must be accompanied by name of affiliated institution, date of term, and the *signature* of program/residency coordinator on institution letterhead. Orders will be billed at individual rate until proof of status is received. Foreign air speed delivery is included in all *Clinics* subscription prices. All prices are subject to change without notice. **POSTMASTER:** Send address change to *Gastrointestinal Endoscopy Clinics of North America*, Elsevier Health Sciences Division, Subscription Customer Service, 3251 Riverport Lane, Maryland Heights, MO 63043. **Customer Service: 1-800-654-2452 (US). From outside the United States, call 1-314-447-8871. Fax: 1-314-447-8029. E-mail: JournalsCustomerService-usa@elsevier.com (for print support) or JournalsOnlineSupport-usa@elsevier.com (for online support).**

Reprints. For copies of 100 or more, of articles in this publication, please contact the Commercial Reprints Department, Elsevier Inc., 360 Park Avenue South, New York, NY 10010-1710. Tel. 212-633-3874; Fax: 212-633-3820; E-mail: reprints@elsevier.com.

Gastrointestinal Endoscopy Clinics of North America is covered in *Excerpta Medica, MEDLINE/PubMed (Index Medicus), and MEDLINE/MEDLARS.*

Contributors

CONSULTING EDITOR

CHARLES J. LIGHTDALE, MD
Professor of Medicine, Division of Digestive and Liver Diseases, Columbia University Medical Center, New York, New York, USA

EDITORS

ROY SOETIKNO, MD, MS (Health Services Research), MSM, FASGE
Advanced Gastrointestinal Endoscopy, Mountain View, California, USA; Advanced Gastrointestinal Endoscopy, Palo Alto, California, USA; The University of Indonesia, Jakarta, Indonesia

TONYA KALTENBACH, MD, MS (Clinical Research)
Advanced Gastrointestinal Endoscopy, Mountain View, California, USA; Associate Professor of Clinical Medicine, Division of Gastroenterology and Hepatology, University of California, San Francisco, Department of Gastroenterology, San Francisco Veterans Affairs Medical Center, Veterans Affairs San Francisco Healthcare System, San Francisco, California, USA

AUTHORS

MAJIDAH ABDULFATTAH BUKHARI, MD, FASGE, FRCPC, ABIM, MRCP (GI)
Consultant, Gastroenterologist and Hepatologist, Advanced Therapeutic Endoscopist, Gastrointestinal Motility, Division of Gastroenterology and Hepatology, Johns Hopkins Medical Institutions, Baltimore, Maryland, USA; Division of Medicine and Gastroenterology and Hepatology International Medical Center in Jeddah, Saudi Arabia

RAVISHANKAR ASOKKUMAR, MBBS, MD, MRCP
Bariatric Endoscopy Unit, HM Sanchinarro University Hospital, Madrid, Spain; Department of Gastroenterology and Hepatology, Singapore General Hospital, Singapore, Singapore

MOHAN PAPPU BABU, MD
Department of Internal Medicine, University of Arizona, Banner University Medical Center, Tucson, Arizona, USA

INMACULADA BAUTISTA, MD, PhD
Bariatric Endoscopy Unit, HM Sanchinarro University Hospital, Madrid, Spain

KAREL CACA, MD, PhD
Department of Gastroenterology and Oncology, Klinikum Ludwigsburg, Ludwigsburg, Germany

JASON CHANG PIK EU, MD
Department of Gastroenterology and Hepatology, Singapore General Hospital, Singapore

YUNG-KA CHIN, MD, MBChB, MRCP
Department of Gastroenterology and Hepatology, Singapore General Hospital, Singapore

PHILLIP S. GE, MD
Assistant Professor, Department of Gastroenterology, Hepatology and Nutrition, The University of Texas MD Anderson Cancer Center, Houston, Texas, USA

NICOLAS GLASER, MD
Department of Medicine II, Faculty of Medicine, University of Freiburg, Medical Centre, Freiburg, Germany

HAZEM HAMMAD, MD
Division of Gastroenterology and Hepatology, University of Colorado Hospital, Anschutz Medical Campus, University of Colorado, Aurora, Colorado, USA

DIEGO JUZGADO, MD
Head of Department, Gastroenterology Department, Hospital Quironsalud Madrid, Madrid, Spain

TONYA KALTENBACH, MD, MS (Clinical Research)
Advanced Gastrointestinal Endoscopy, Mountain View, California, USA; Associate Professor of Clinical Medicine, Division of Gastroenterology and Hepatology, University of California, San Francisco, Department of Gastroenterology, San Francisco Veterans Affairs Medical Center, Veterans Affairs San Francisco Healthcare System, San Francisco, California, USA

SERGEY V. KANTSEVOY, MD, PhD
Director of Therapeutic Endoscopy, Mercy Medical Center, Baltimore, Maryland, USA

MOUEN A. KHASHAB, MD
Associate Professor of Medicine, Division of Gastroenterology and Hepatology, Johns Hopkins Medical Institutions, Division of Gastroenterology and Hepatology, Johns Hopkins Hospital, Baltimore, Maryland, USA

JENNIFER M. KOLB, MD
Division of Gastroenterology and Hepatology, University of Colorado Hospital, Anschutz Medical Campus, University of Colorado, Aurora, Colorado, USA

THOMAS KRATT, MD
Department of Surgery, University of Heidelberg, Heidelberg, Germany

ARMIN KUELLMER, MD
Department of Medicine II, Faculty of Medicine, University of Freiburg, Medical Centre, Freiburg, Germany

JAMES LAU, MD, PhD
Department of Surgery, Prince of Wales Hospital, Shatin, NT, Hong Kong SAR

GONTRAND LOPEZ-NAVA, MD, PhD, FASGE
Bariatric Endoscopy Unit, HM Sanchinarro University Hospital, Madrid, Spain

CARMEL MALVAR, BA
Section of Gastroenterology, San Francisco Veterans Affairs Medical Center, Division of Gastroenterology and Hepatology, University of California, San Francisco, San Francisco, California, USA

ALVARO MARTÍNEZ-ALCALÁ, MD
Department of Gastroenterology, Hospital Universitario Infanta Leonor, Madrid, Spain

PARIT MEKAROONKAMOL, MD
Division of Gastroenterology, Faculty of Medicine, Chulalongkorn University, King Chulalongkorn Memorial Hospital, Bangkok, Thailand

KLAUS MÖNKEMÜLLER, MD, PhD, FASGE
Department of Gastroenterology, Helios Frankenwaldklinik, Kronach, Germany; Department of Gastroenterology, Otto-von-Guericke University, Magdeburg, Germany; University of Belgrade, Belgrade, Serbia

TIFFANY NGUYEN-VU, BA
Department of Gastroenterology, San Francisco Veterans Affairs Medical Center, San Francisco, California, USA

PANIDA PIYACHATURAWAT, MD
Division of Gastroenterology, Faculty of Medicine, Chulalongkorn University, King Chulalongkorn Memorial Hospital, Bangkok, Thailand

RUNGSUN RERKNIMITR, MD
Division of Gastroenterology, Faculty of Medicine, Chulalongkorn University, King Chulalongkorn Memorial Hospital, Bangkok, Thailand

W. ALTON RUSSELL, MS
Department of Management Sciences and Engineering, Stanford University, Stanford, California, USA

ENNALIZA SALAZAR, MD
Department of Gastroenterology and Hepatology, Singapore General Hospital, Singapore

ANDRES SANCHEZ-YAGUE, MD, PhD, FACG, FASGE
Head of Department, Gastroenterology Department, Vithas Xanit International Hospital, Benalmadena, Spain; Interventional Endoscopy, Gastroenterology Department, Hospital Costa del Sol, Marbella, Spain

SILVIA SANDULEANU, MD, PhD
Division of Gastroenterology and Hepatology, Maastricht University Medical Center, Maastricht, The Netherlands

ARTHUR R. SCHMIDT, MD, PhD
Department of Medicine II, Faculty of Medicine, Division of Interdisciplinary Endoscopy, University of Freiburg, Medical Centre, Freiburg, Germany

ALLISON R. SCHULMAN MD, MPH
Division of Gastroenterology and Hepatology, University of Michigan, Ann Arbor, Michigan, USA

ROY SOETIKNO, MD, MS (Health Services Research), MSM, FASGE
Advanced Gastrointestinal Endoscopy, Mountain View, California, USA; Advanced GI Endoscopy, Palo Alto, California, USA; The University of Indonesia, Jakarta, Indonesia

CHRISTOPHER C. THOMPSON, MD, MSc, FACG, FASGE, AGAF
Associate Professor, Division of Gastroenterology, Hepatology and Endoscopy, Brigham and Women's Hospital, Boston, Massachusetts, USA

RABINDRA R. WATSON, MD, FASGE
Director of Bariatric Endoscopy, Interventional Endoscopy Services, California Pacific Medical Center, Associate Clinical Professor of Medicine, University of California, San Francisco, San Francisco, California, USA

JESSICA X. YU, MD, MS
Division of Gastroenterology and Hepatology, University of Michigan, Ann Arbor, Michigan, USA

Contents

 Video content accompanies this article at http://www.giendo. theclinics.com.

The over the scope clip is a novel endoscopic tool developed for tissue compression in the gastrointestinal tract. It has already revolutionized the management of acute perforations and leaks. In the past decade, it has also increasingly been used for treatment of severe and/or refractory gastrointestinal hemorrhage. Available studies report high rates of primary hemostasis and rebleeding. This article provides an overview on available literature, potential indications, and technical aspects of hemostasis with over the scope clip.

Endoscopic treatment of lower gastrointestinal bleeding can be challenging. This article reports on the use of the endoscopic clipping over the scope technique to treat acute severe lower gastrointestinal bleeding. In particular, it describes the approaches and outcomes of using the technique for acute severe bleeding in the colon and the anal transition zone. The following synopsis is the one that you supplied, but lightly copyedited. Please confirm OK. Please note that the synopsis will appear in PubMed: Endoscopic treatment of lower gastrointestinal bleeding can be challenging. This article reports on the use of the endoscopic clipping over the scope technique to treat acute severe lower gastrointestinal bleeding. In particular, it describes the approaches and outcomes of using the technique for acute severe bleeding in the colon and the anal transition zone.

 Video content accompanies this article at http://www.giendo. theclinics.com.

In gastrointestinal perforation or fistula, endoscopic closure techniques could be used as alternatives to surgery. Early endoscopic recognition and treatment of gastrointestinal perforation is the most important factor determining procedural success and clinical outcomes. The over the scope clip with full-thickness grasping capability provides greater technical and clinical success rates compared with the through the scope clips. Although the technical success rate of chronic fistula closure is comparable to perforation closure, it has a significantly lower clinical success owing to its less healthy tissue edge of the fistula. The over the scope clip system should be considered before surgery for the closure of perforation and fistula.

   Video content accompanies this article at http://www.giendo. theclinics.com.

Despite major improvements in endoscopic devices and therapeutic endoscopy, closure of gastrointestinal perforations, dehiscence, and fistulae had remained problematic. However, since the advent of devices such as the over the scope clip and others, endoscopic closure of gastrointestinal defects has become a routine approach. Furthermore, because of its strong apposition force, the over the scope clip may also be used to anchor fully covered self-expanding metal stents. In addition, the over the scope clip is an effective rescue therapy for various types of gastrointestinal bleeding pathologies. It is frequently used as an additional tool in complex gastrointestinal leak cases requiring internal and external drains.

The over the scope clip is safe and efficacious and has become the preferred device of choice for the treatment of complex gastrointestinal bleeding, perforation, and gastrointestinal leaks. With its widespread adoption in clinical practice, information on complications associated with over the scope clip use is emerging. Nonetheless, the overall complication rate is still very low. Most of the reported complications have been related to the technique rather than the actual device and could likely be prevented with proper technique. In this article, the authors summarize the complications associated with over the scope clip use and provide guidance on safety measure to mitigate them.

Clipping over the scope (C-OTS) is a novel closure technique used for the treatment of nonvariceal gastrointestinal bleeding, especially for high-risk lesions. C-OTS devices cost more than clipping through the scope and thermal devices. The high upfront cost of C-OTS may pose a barrier to its use and the cost-effectiveness of C-OTS for peptic ulcer disease bleeding is unknown. Cost-effectiveness studies of C-OTS for peptic ulcer bleeding as both first-line and second-line therapy can provide the current estimate of the conditions in which the use of C-OTS is cost-effective and give insights of the determinants to the cost-effectiveness of C-OTS.

Training practicing physicians to adopt new technology may be difficult because most endoscopy training is given during fellowship training. As such, the adoption of new technology in gastroenterology is typically slow. We designed our course to train our cohort of practicing physicians using flipped learning, a pedagogical approach in which instructional cognitive content is delivered to the individual instead of the group, usually through online platforms and outside of the classroom. We describe our methods and results of the training courses on the techniques of clipping over the scope for gastrointestinal bleeding and endoscopic balloon dilation.

Endoscopic suturing device for flexible endoscopy was conceptualized by Apollo Group in collaboration with Olympus Optical Ltd. The first modification of suturing device for flexible endoscopy (Eagle Claw) was manufactured by Olympus engineers and extensively used by members of Apollo Group in numerous bench-top experiments on isolated pig stomachs and in live porcine model. The suturing system for flexible endoscopy in humans (Overstitch) was cleared for general clinical use in the United States in 2008. The latest model is compatible with more than 20 single-channel flexible endoscopes with diameters ranging from 8.8 mm to 9.8 mm made by major endoscope manufacturers.

 Video content accompanies this article at http://www.giendo. theclinics.com.

Obesity is a public health pandemic and leading contributor to morbidity and mortality. Endoscopic bariatric therapies have emerged as a viable minimally invasive treatment option to fill the therapeutic gap between conservative and surgical approaches. The ability to reliably place full-thickness sutures throughout the gastrointestinal tract has opened the door to novel endoscopic gastric restrictive procedures. A growing body of literature supports endoscopic sleeve gastroplasty as a safe, effective, and reproducible endoscopic treatment of obesity and metabolic syndrome. In addition, endoscopic sutured revision procedures following gastric bypass and sleeve gastrectomy are now first-line with demonstrable safety and long-term efficacy.

important to understand suture patterns and the different traction methods available. Applications beyond tissue compression in bariatric endoscopy include: closure, traction and fixation. Closure could be applied to perforations, suture dehiscences, fistulas and stoma reduction. Traction could be applied either as a pulley method to improver resection or as an improved method to decrease a defect size and help pull it into an over the scope clip. Fixation has been mainly used to secure stents.

Jessica X. Yu and Allison R. Schulman

Endoscopic suturing with the OverStitch device is safe and effective for a wide range of applications from defect closure and stent fixation to hemostasis and bariatrics. OverStitch-related complications remain rare, although adverse events such as bleeding, mucosal injury, perigastric fluid collections, leaks, and perforations have been reported. Provider familiarity with the device and the specific pitfalls that may arise with OverStitch use in different situations is necessary to minimize the risk of adverse events. This article reviews potential complications and provides tips and troubleshooting techniques.

Majidah Abdulfattah Bukhari and Mouen A. Khashab

Successful closure of gastrointestinal defects is one of the most important goals for therapeutic endoscopy. Historically, surgical repair was the mainstay of treatment for any gastrointestinal defect; however, surgery is associated with high morbidity and mortality. Endoscopic management of gastrointestinal defects has developed rapidly in recent years and has become more effective, reducing the morbidity and mortality rates, and avoiding surgical interventions. Appropriate use of endoscopic techniques requires extensive knowledge of the devices and their advantages and limitations during practical applications.

GASTROINTESTINAL ENDOSCOPY CLINICS OF NORTH AMERICA

RELATED CLINICS SERIES

Gastroenterology Clinics
Clinics in Liver Disease

THE CLINICS ARE AVAILABLE ONLINE!
Access your subscription at:
www.theclinics.com

Foreword

Closure Power: Advances in Endoscopic Clipping and Sewing

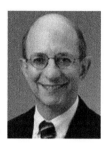

Charles J. Lightdale, MD
Consulting Editor

Gastrointestinal endoscopists have long been called one-handed surgeons. Through the scope channels allowed the passage of instruments that were excellent for injection, resection, cauterization, and tissue retrieval. Think of the essential cautery snare, the Roth net, and more recently, the needle knife and the coagulation grasper. However, even with competitive improvements, through the scope clips often lacked critical size and strength to close a perforation or stop an arterial bleed. Sewing, a surgical skill that requires 2 hands or rigid laparoscopic instruments, was available to only a few experts using flexible endoscopes employing early endoscopic sewing devices that were awkward and difficult. Recent advances, however, in over the scope clips and significant improvements in endoscopic sewing machines have brought new power for closure to flexible endoscopy. These advances have already had an impact in expanding the role of flexible endoscopy to close perforations, large resections, and fistulas; to stop bleeding; to secure stents; and to perform new bariatric procedures.

I am particularly pleased that Roy Soetikno and Tonya Kaltenbach have teamed up to be the editors for this issue of *Gastrointestinal Endoscopy Clinics of North America* focused on flexible endoscopic closure techniques of over the scope clipping and sewing. They have tapped into thoughtful and talented national and international experts, who have produced articles with an emphasis on usability and practicality. There are detailed descriptions of technique with pictures on how to use over the scope clips and sutures and how to avoid complications in different clinical situations. Also included are key articles regarding training, and the importance of getting these incredibly effective new methods into more widespread use. Increased closure power is here and available. Open-minded gastrointestinal endoscopists should read this

Gastrointest Endoscopy Clin N Am 30 (2020) xiii–xiv
https://doi.org/10.1016/j.giec.2019.10.002
1052-5157/20/© 2019 Published by Elsevier Inc.

giendo.theclinics.com

issue of *Gastrointestinal Endoscopy Clinics of North America* in its entirety and consider how to bring the benefits of closure power to their practice.

Charles J. Lightdale, MD
Department of Medicine
Columbia University Medical Center
161 Fort Washington Avenue
New York, NY 10032, USA

E-mail address:
CJL18@columbia.edu

Preface

Endoscopic Closure Techniques: Endoscopic Clipping Over the Scope (C-OTS) and Endoscopic Suturing

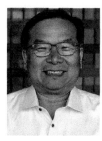 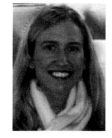

Roy Soetikno, MD   Tonya Kaltenbach, MD
Editors

Over the past 3 decades, significant improvements and innovations have occurred in the field of diagnostic and therapeutic endoscopy. For example, the availability of high-definition endoscopes with detailed image enhancement capabilities allows us to routinely seek out nonpolypoid and precancerous lesions within the gastrointestinal tract; the wide variety of user-friendly accessories allows us to perform more complex resections through the endoscope, and advancements with endoscopic ultrasound allows us to perform precise assessments and therapies. In addition, we are now able to perform complex endobiliary therapies endoscopically. Many of these advancements have replaced the needs for surgery and have allowed us to achieve similar, if not, improved outcomes.

We are indebted to Professor Charlie Lightdale for the opportunity to collate the current knowledge about endoscopic clipping over the scope (C-OTS) and suturing techniques. In addition, we are grateful to all the authors who willingly contributed to this issue despite their busy schedules. We believe that this issue, which discusses the latest developments of C-OTS and suturing techniques, is much needed and important.

We envision that the issue will serve as a review and practical resource guide. As such, this issue contains atlases on C-OTS and suturing techniques. It also includes information on the techniques' cost-effectiveness and training. Earlier this year, through the program announcement 19-065, the National Institutes of Health highlighted the need to further develop simulation technology in order to help improve skill acquisition and maintenance of practicing endoscopy physicians.[1] We thus included

Gastrointest Endoscopy Clin N Am 30 (2020) xv–xvi
https://doi.org/10.1016/j.giec.2019.10.001
1052-5157/20/© 2019 Published by Elsevier Inc.

an article that discusses how to effectively train practicing physicians in new techniques, such as C-OTS, through flipped learning and simulator-based training.

It is important that we standardize our nomenclature for endoscopic clipping techniques. Today, our clipping techniques include over the scope and through the scope devices. In order to be consistent, we believe that the terms endoscopic C-OTS and C-TTS, which refer to over the scope and through the scope, respectively, are necessary as they describe the techniques precisely. Furthermore, these terms help us to avoid confusion between the technique of over the scope clipping and the device Over The Scope Clip (OTSC, Ovesco Endoscopy AG, Tuebingen, Germany), which is trademarked.

Editing an issue on high-tech devices can be challenging because the techniques and data are still evolving. For example, we are still waiting for the results of ongoing studies that evaluate the use of C-OTS as the first-line modality to treat upper gastrointestinal bleeding. Moreover, it is important to note that there are other clips, such as The Padlock(US Endoscopy, Mentor, OH, USA) clips, that are deployed over the scope. However, due to the lack of literature on this technology, we could not discuss it extensively in this issue.

Looking over the horizon, the future of endoscopy appears to be very bright and expansive. There are, however, some challenges that we must overcome in order to make our progress more widespread. Among the more pressing challenges is the need to train our current trainees more efficiently and effectively. Similarly, we need to provide our practicing endoscopists with opportunities to continuously train and acquire new knowledge and skills. In short, we need to revolutionize the way we train and retrain endoscopy so that we can achieve the true potential of endoscopy.

Roy Soetikno, MD
Advanced Gastrointestinal Endoscopy
2490 Hospital Drive
Mountain View, CA 94040, USA

Tonya Kaltenbach, MD
Division of Gastroenterology
University of California, San Francisco
San Francisco, CA 94121, USA

E-mail addresses:
Soetikno@earthlink.net (R. Soetikno)
endoresection@me.com (T. Kaltenbach)

REFERENCE

1. PA-19-065: Medical simulators for practicing patient care providers skill acquisition, outcomes assessment and technology development (R01 Clinical Trial Not Allowed). Available at: https://grants.nih.gov/grants/guide/pa-files/PA-19-065.html. Accessed August 29, 2019.

The Use of the Over the Scope Clip to Treat Upper Gastrointestinal Bleeding

Arthur R. Schmidt, MD, PhD[a],*, Nicolas Glaser, MD[a],
Armin Kuellmer, MD[a], Karel Caca, MD, PhD[b], James Lau, MD, PhD[c]

KEYWORDS

- Over the scope clip • UGIB • Bleeding • Hemostasis

KEY POINTS

- The over the scope clip (OTSC) is a novel tool developed for tissue compression in the gastrointestinal tract.
- Apart from closure of perforations and leaks, available studies also suggest high efficacy for endoscopic treatment of upper gastrointestinal bleeding.
- Compared to conventional through the scope clips, OTSC are able to grasp a larger amount of tissue, exhibit higher compression force and allow effective anchoring in fibrotic tissue.
- Apart from recurrent peptic ulcer bleeding, OTSC may be used as first-line therapy for patients at high risk of rebleeding.
- This review gives an overview on available literature, potential indications, and technical aspects of hemostasis with OTSC.

 Video content accompanies this article at http://www.giendo.theclinics.com.

INTRODUCTION

Upper gastrointestinal bleeding (UGIB) is one of the leading causes of hospital admission with substantial economic impact. The incidence of hospitalization related to acute UGIB was reported as 66 cases per 100,000.[1] Despite advances in medical

Conflicts of Interest: A. Schmidt and K. Caca received lecture fees and study grants from Ovesco Endoscopy. J. Lau received lecture fees from Boston Scientific, Cook, and Olympus companies.
[a] Department of Medicine II, Faculty of Medicine, University of Freiburg, Medical Centre, Freiburg, Germany; [b] Department of Gastroenterology and Oncology, Klinikum Ludwigsburg, Posilipostraße 4, Ludwigsburg 71640, Germany; [c] Department of Surgery, Prince of Wales Hospital, 30-32 Ngan Shing Street, Shatin, NT, Hong Kong SAR
* Correspondence author. Department of Medicine II, Faculty of Medicine, University of Freiburg, Medical Centre, Hugstetter Strasse 55, Freiburg 79160, Germany.
E-mail address: arthur.schmidt@uniklinik-freiburg.de

Gastrointest Endoscopy Clin N Am 30 (2020) 1–11
https://doi.org/10.1016/j.giec.2019.08.001
1052-5157/20/© 2019 Elsevier Inc. All rights reserved.

and interventional treatment, management of severe bleeding remains challenging and mortality of acute peptic ulcer bleeding (PUB) amounts up to 8.6%.[2,3] Endoscopic hemostasis was shown to reduce mortality, need for blood transfusion, and surgery and is therefore the mainstay of therapy. Through the scope clips or thermal therapy with or without combination injection of adrenaline solution are considered standard endoscopic treatment.[4] Although hemostasis with standard methods is successful in about 90% of cases, treatment failure remains a major concern. Rebleeding was shown to be a predictor of increased mortality and success rates of endoscopic retreatment with standard methods drop to around 75%.[5] However, surgical salvage therapy is associated with mortality rates up to 29%.[6] Hence, primary durable control of bleeding is mandatory and there is a need to improve endoscopic therapy, especially for patients at high risk of treatment failure. The over the scope clip (over the scope clip, Ovesco Endoscopy, Tuebingen, Germany) is a novel endoscopic tool developed for tissue compression in the gastrointestinal (GI) tract. It has already revolutionized the management of acute perforations and leaks. In the past decade, it has also increasingly been used for treatment of severe and/or refractory GI hemorrhage. This review gives an overview on available literature and focuses on technical aspects of hemostasis with over the scope clip (Videos 1–4).

PUBLISHED DATA ON TREATMENT OF UPPER GASTROINTESTINAL BLEEDING WITH OVER THE SCOPE CLIP

Since the introduction of the over the scope clip system in 2006, many groups have reported their experience on treatment of UGIB.[7–11] Apart from initial case reports and small single-center series, there are now several retrospective multicenter studies reporting on greater than 100 cases. To date, only one randomized controlled trial comparing over the scope clip with standard treatment has been published.[12]

One of the first reports on over the scope clip hemostasis in UGIB was published in 2011 by Kirschniak and colleagues[13] including 12 cases. Primary hemostasis was achieved in all cases with a rebleeding rate of 17%. Manta and colleagues[14] reported a larger series in 2013 of 23 cases with UGIB refractory to standard endoscopic treatment, most of them being duodenal and gastric ulcers. Primary hemostasis was achieved in 22 of 23 cases (95.7%) and rebleeding occurred in only two patients (9.0%). Two years later, Manno and colleagues[15] reported 100% technical success with no rebleeding in 40 consecutive patients with UGIB using over the scope clip as the first-line treatment. In the same year, Wedi and colleagues[16] published a similar retrospective study including 41 patients with UGIB, mostly from gastroduodenal ulcers. In 31.7% over the scope clip was used as second-line therapy and clinical success was achieved in 85.4%. Richter-Schrag and colleagues[17] reported on a single-center cohort of 100 cases, including 69 patients with UGIB. Primary hemostasis and clinical success were achieved in 88% and 78%, respectively. This study also compared over the scope clip as first-line versus second-line endoscopic therapy (FLET vs SLET). Technical failure and rebleeding rates were significantly higher in the SLET versus the FLET group (8.2% vs 4.9% and 28.2% vs 23.1%). This was not unexpected because patients who failed conventional therapy may represent a cohort at higher risk of rebleeding. Those with a Rockall Score greater than seven had significantly lower rates of rebleeding when treated with over the scope clip. Another retrospective study reported on over the scope clip hemostasis in 75 patients, most of them under antithrombotic therapy. Sixty-five of 75 patients had bleeding from gastroduodenal ulcers.[18] Immediate hemostasis was achieved in all cases and rebleeding occurred in 34.7%, predominantly in patients with antiplatelet agents. However, all but three patients could be further treated endoscopically without need for surgery or angiographic embolization. The authors concluded that over the scope clip should be the primary treatment of choice in this critically ill patient population.

The FLET ROCK study by Wedi and colleagues[19] investigated mortality and rebleeding rates of 117 patients treated with over the scope clip from three centers. Results of this cohort were compared with predicted rates by the Rockall score. Compared with Rockall prediction, mortality after rebleeding was significantly reduced from 27.9% to 10.9% in the high-risk group (Rockall score ≥8) treated with FLET. Furthermore, the occurrence of rebleeding or continued bleeding was significantly lower in the moderate-risk group (Rockall score 4–7) and in the high-risk group (Rockall score ≥8) compared with the Rockall cohort, respectively (P<.001). Although this study has methodologic weaknesses (retrospective data collection and comparison with historical cohort) it strongly suggests that over the scope clip first-line treatment may improve prognosis of high-risk patients.

A recent study by Brandler and colleagues[20] investigated over the scope clip first-line (n = 49) and second-line (n = 18) treatment in high-risk lesions. Definition of high-risk lesions was: location in the area of a major artery and larger than 20 mm in diameter and/or a deep penetrating, excavated, fibrotic ulcer with high-risk stigmata, or lesions that could not be treated by standard endoscopy. Similar to other studies previously described, total success rate in this high-risk cohort was 81.3%, respectively.

The largest series available to date was recently published by Manta and colleagues.[21] In this retrospective multicenter Italian study, over the scope clip were applied in 286 patients, most (n = 214) with UGIB. over the scope clip was used as first-line therapy in lesions classified as high risk. Results were favorable with a reported primary hemostasis rate of 96.4% and a rebleeding rate of only 4.4%. **Table 1** shows an overview of available studies including greater than 10 patients.

Taken together, all studies mentioned indicate high efficacy of over the scope clip hemostasis (**Table 1**). However, these retrospective cohort studies included heterogenous patients with varying source and severity of bleeding. over the scope clips were used as primary and rescue therapy. The only prospective randomized trial available to date is the STING (STop bleedING) study.[12] This multicenter study included patients with recurrent bleeding from peptic gastroduodenal ulcers after initial endoscopic hemostasis. Sixty-six patients were randomized to over the scope clip versus standard endoscopic treatment. The latter was defined as through the scope (TTS) clip or thermal therapy plus injection of adrenaline solution. Clinical success (absence of persistent or recurrent bleeding) was significantly higher in the over the scope clip versus the standard therapy group (84.8% vs 42.4%; P = .001). However, no significant difference in mortality or need for surgical or angiographic therapy was observed. This may be caused by the low number of patients included and by the crossover design of the study. A prospective multicenter trial on over the scope clip first-line treatment in patients at high risk for rebleeding is already recruiting and first results are expected in the near future (clinicaltrials.gov NCT03331224).

LIMITATIONS OF CONVENTIONAL ENDOSCOPIC METHODS AND POTENTIAL INDICATIONS FOR HEMOSTASIS WITH OVER THE SCOPE CLIP

Thermal or mechanical clip treatment with or without injection therapy are the recommended gold standard therapies for endoscopic hemostasis.[4] However, these methods have several limitations. Thermal treatment is associated with risk of transmural injury and perforation, especially in case of deep excavated ulcers. In an

Table 1
Overview of available studies including greater than 10 cases on over the scope clip hemostasis

Author, Year	Type of Study	N	Therapy	Bleeding Source	Primary Success (%)	Rebleeding (%)	Clinical Success (%)
Kirschniak et al,[13] 2011	Retrospective	12	1st line	Various	12/12 (100)	2/12 (17)	10/12 (83)
Manta et al,[14] 2013	Retrospective, multicenter	30	2nd line	Various	29/30 (97)	2/30 (7)	27/30 (90)
Skinner et al,[25] 2014	Retrospective, single center	12	2nd line	Various	12/12 (100)	2/12 (17)	10/12 (83)
Manno et al,[15] 2016	Retrospective, single center	40	1st line	Various	40/40 (100)	0	40/40 (100)
Richter-Schrag et al,[17] 2016	Retrospective, single center	63	1st line and 2nd line	Various	54/63 (86)	11/63 (16)	43/63 (68)
Wedi et al,[16] 2016	Retrospective, single center	41	1st line and 2nd line	Various	35/41 (85)	6/41 (15)	35/41 (85)
Honegger et al,[7] 2017	Retrospective, single center	53	1st line	Various	48/53 (91)	7/53 (13)	41/53 (77)
Kobara et al,[9] 2017	Retrospective, multicenter	18	2nd line	Various	16/18 (89)	1/18 (6)	15/18 (83)
Lamberts et al,[18] 2017	Retrospective, single center	68	1st line and 2nd line	Various	68/68 (100)	24 (35)	44 (65)
Brandler et al,[20] 2018	Retrospective, single-center	67	1st line and 2nd line	Various (high-risk lesions)	n/a	9/67 (13)	47/67 (70.1)
Wedi et al,[11] 2017	Retrospective, two centers	100	1st line and 2nd line	Various	94/100 (94)	8/100 (8)	86/100 (86)
Wedi et al,[19] 2018	Retrospective, multicenter, comparison with Rockall cohort	118	1st line	Various	109/118 (93)	16/118 (13)	93/118 (79)
Schmidt et al,[12] 2018	RCT, multicenter	66 (33 vs 33)	2nd line	Gastroduodenal peptic ulcers	31/33 (93.9)	3/33 (9.1)	28/33 (84%; 8)
Manta et al,[21] 2018	Retrospective, multicenter	214	1st line	Various	202/2014 (97)	9 (4%; 5)	193 (90)
Asokkumar et al,[10] 2018	Retrospective, single center	18	1st line and 2nd line	Various	18/18 (100)	0 (0)	18/18 (100)
Pooled analysis		820			768/820 (93%; 7)	100/820 (12%; 1)	730/820 (89%; 0)

Abbreviations: n/a, not available; RCT, randomized controlled trial.
The number of patients (n) refers only to patients with UGIB within in the study. Primary success is defined as immediate hemostasis by over the scope clip. Clinical success is defined as durable hemostasis with absence of rebleeding.

ex vivo model, endoscopic thermocoagulation could only consistently seal arteries up to 2 mm.[22,23] TTS clips are difficult to apply in locations like the duodenal bulb and in the fibrotic tissue of large ulcers. Even if clip application is possible in those cases, they tend to dislodge prematurely leading to recurrent bleeding.

Compared with conventional hemostatic methods, over the scope clip have the following advantages:

- Ability to grasp a larger amount of tissue
- Higher compression force[24]
- More effective anchoring in fibrotic tissue
- Applicator cap allows better visualization of the bleeding source and facilitates clip placement in narrow or difficult-to-access anatomic sites[8,25]
- Low rate of clip-related complication rate
- High rate of clip retention

However, because of the lack of prospective trials, indications for hemostasis with over the scope clip are not well defined. The current European Society of Gastrointestinal Endoscopy guideline, which was published in 2016, recommends over the scope clip treatment "when bleeding is refractory or not amenable to standard endoscopic hemostasis therapies."[4] For recurrent PUB, the STING study demonstrated clear superiority of over the scope clip when compared with TTS clips + injection therapy. Therefore, over the scope clip can be recommended as a rescue therapy for refractory PUB. For first-line therapy, there is currently no published prospective comparative trial. However, existing retrospective data on large patient cohorts suggest favorable efficacy in patients with high risk of treatment failure.

Therefore, we suggest hemostasis with over the scope clip for second-line therapy in patients with recurrent or persistent bleeding from gastroduodenal ulcers after failure of conventional endoscopic methods (high level of evidence). First-line over the scope clip therapy may be considered in patients with high risk of treatment failure (low evidence, prospective studies lacking):

- Large fibrotic ulcers ($\geq$2 cm)
- Bleeding sites difficult to access (eg, posterior wall of duodenal bulb or gastric lesser curve)
- Patients on continued anticoagulants and/or dual antiplatelet therapy
- Other factors associated with high risk of rebleeding may also be considered (comorbidities, hemodynamic instability, presence of active bleeding, high Rockall score)

TECHNICAL CONSIDERATIONS, TIPS, AND TRICKS FOR CLINICAL PRACTICE
The Over the Scope Clip System

The over the scope clip is a super elastic nitinol clip that was developed for tissue approximation and compression in the digestive tract. Because of the memory effect of the nitinol, the clip closes after it is released from the applicator cap and then delivers constant force to the tissue. The clips are bio- and MRI-compatible and can remain in vivo as long-term implants.

The applicator cap comes in two different depths (3 mm and 6 mm). The 6-mm cap can capture more tissue and is the standard cap for perforation closure. We also use the 6-mm cap for hemostasis in nearly all cases. However, the 3-mm cap may also be used, especially for fibrotic ulcers or narrow anatomic spaces.

The clip is available in three different designs and four sizes (**Fig. 1**). The type-a clip has blunt teeth and is primarily intended for tissue compression. The teeth of the type-t

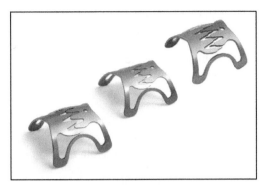

Fig. 1. Types of Over the Scope clip. Three different types are available: type "a" (*left*), type "t" (*middle*), and type "gc" (*right*). (*Courtesy of* Ovesco Endoscopy, Tuebingen, Germany; with permission.)

clip exhibit small spikes that are supposed to enhance the anchoring effect. The type-gc clip is primarily intended for closure of gastric perforations. For hemostasis in the upper GI tract we generally prefer the type-t clip, especially for fibrotic ulcers because we believe that the anchoring effect is important for effective hemostasis in these cases. However, many groups also use the type-a variant; comparative studies do not exist. All clip variants come in 11-, 12-, and 14-mm diameter. The 11- and 12-mm devices are used with endoscopes with an outer diameter of 8.5 mm to 12 mm, whereas the 14-mm clips are intended for use with a 10.5- to 12-mm endoscope. In our experience the 12-mm clip is suitable for nearly all cases; we use the 12/6t as standard device in upper GI hemostasis. If passage through the upper esophageal sphincter or through the pylorus is difficult, the 11-mm clip may be used instead of the 12-mm version. There is also a novel "mini over the scope clip" system (10-mm diameter) that is intended to facilitate treatment in small lumen (eg, children) or in other difficult-to-access sites. However, we have no experience with this novel system.

Hemostasis with Over the Scope Clip: Step-by-Step

Hemostasis with over the scope clip is generally a simple procedure, which might even be easier to learn compared with TTS clip application. However, correct clip positioning is crucial because retreatment might be difficult in case of misplacement.

The steps of over the scope clip hemostasis are as follows:

1. Identification of bleeding source: Before assembly of the over the scope clip system, the bleeding source should be identified and assessed endoscopically. In case of active bleeding, we generally do not use epinephrine injection before clip placement because this may hamper immediate evaluation of treatment success after clip application. However, in case of severe bleeding, prior injection therapy may help to improve visualization of the bleeding vessel.
2. over the scope clip assembly: Hemostasis using over the scope clip is often an emergency procedure. The team should be familiar with assembly of the system, which is similar to that of a ligation device. First, the handwheel is mounted on the working channel of the endoscope. The thread retriever is then used to pull the thread through the working channel. The thread is then passed into the gap of the handwheel and winded up with the wheel. The applicator cap is then mounted on the tip of the endoscope. It is important to ensure that the tip of the

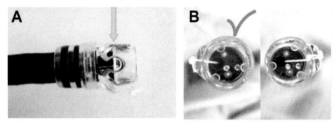

Fig. 2. Assembly of the Over the Scope clip system. It is important to ensure that the tip of the cap reaches the stoppers/marking (arrow) in the cap (*A*) and that the thread does not impair vision and runs straight in the working channel (*B*). (*Courtesy of* Ovesco Endoscopy, Tuebingen, Germany.)

cap reaches the stoppers/marking in the cap and that the thread does not impair vision and runs straight in the working channel (**Fig. 2**).

3. Clip placement: The endoscope with the over the scope clip is advanced to the bleeding source. The applicator is advanced until the tip has contact with the tissue of bleeding site. The bleeding vessel/source should be visible in the center of the cap. In case of active bleeding, repeated irrigation using an endo-washer is helpful to improve visualization. The target tissue is then incorporated into the cap only by suction. The use of additional devices, such as anchor, forceps, or twin grasper, is generally not necessary, although may provide more precision to capture the target tissue in cases of severe fibrosis. During suction, it is important to keep the bleeding vessel centrally in the cap. If the tissue slips away laterally, suction should be stopped and the cap should be repositioned. If correct position is ensured, suction is again applied and the over the scope clip is then released from cap by turning the handwheel in a forward direction under continuous suction. Successful release of the clip often cannot be seen during the procedure. Therefore, it is important to turn the handwheel sufficiently in forward direction (sometimes a slight "click" in the wheel is felt after clip release).

4. Inspection of bleeding site: After clip release, suction is stopped and the endoscope is slightly withdrawn to visualize the bleeding site. Correct over the scope clip position (bleeding vessel centrally in the clip) and treatment success (cessation of bleeding or absence of pulsation in an artery) should be carefully assessed.

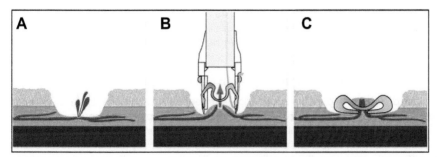

Fig. 3. Schematic illustration of Over the Scope clip application in large fibrotic ulcers. (*A*) Deep ulcer with spurting vessel. (*B*) The cap is placed centrally into the ulcer ground and the tissue is sucked into the cap. (*C*) The Over the Scope clip was placed centrally into the ulcer ground and compressed the central vessel. (*Courtesy of* Ovesco Endoscopy, Tuebingen, Germany.)

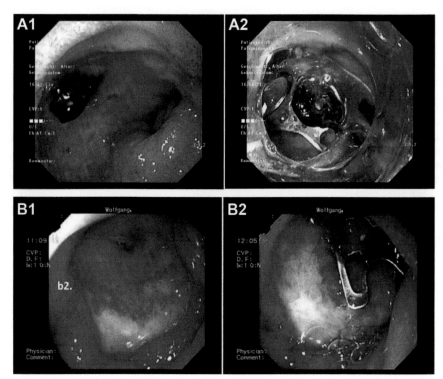

Fig. 4. Examples of two large fibrotic ulcers in the duodenal bulb with central vessel (*A1, B1*). In both cases, the Over the Scope clip was placed in the center of the ulcer ground and was able to effectively compress the vessel (*A2, B2*). (*Courtesy of* Ovesco Endoscopy, Tuebingen, Germany.)

Over the Scope Clip Application in Large Fibrotic Ulcers

In case of small bleeding sources (eg, small ulcers, Dieulafoy lesions) the whole lesion can be sucked into the cap. For large fibrotic ulcers, it is not possible to "close" the whole lesion with the clip; moreover, tissue aspiration into the cap is difficult. In those lesions, the over the scope clip is generally placed onto the ulcer floor grasping the bleeding vessel (**Figs. 3** and **4**). In this situation tissue incorporation may be difficult. It is generally sufficient to just aspirate in as much tissue as possible. Because of its anchoring capabilities, the over the scope clip will still grasp enough tissue to sufficiently compress the bleeding vessel. We recommend to use the type-t clip, which may facilitate anchoring in fibrotic tissue.

How to Proceed When Over the Scope Clip Hemostasis Fails

A major drawback of over the scope clip treatment is that additional endoscopic interventions in case of treatment failure may be hampered by the presence of the large clip. Persistent bleeding or rebleeding generally occurs when the clip is placed laterally to the bleeding vessel or the clip is placed too superficially and is therefore not able to sufficiently compress the bleeding vessel. There are no sufficient data on retreatment after over the scope clip failure and the recommendations given next are therefore based on personal experience:

In case of slight or moderate bleeding, injection of fibrin glue at the lateral border or underneath the clip is attempted. We do not recommend use of thermal therapy because there may be a risk of perforation caused by energy delivery to the disuse underneath the clip. Another possibility of adjunct treatment in the presence of an over the scope clip may be application of a hemostatic powder or gel. Application of TTS clips beneath or even underneath the over the scope clip may also be considered. For severe persistent or recurrent bleeding, endoscopic removal of the clip should be considered. In case of large fibrotic ulcers, the clip generally can grasp little amount of tissue and usually be removed just by pulling with a forceps. After clip removal, a second over the scope clip can be deployed or an alternative hemostatic method attempted. If the clip grasps too much tissue, removal with the forceps might not be possible. Theoretically, a bipolar cutting device (remOVE System, Ovesco Endoscopy) might be used in this case to disintegrate and remove the clip.[26,27] However, this is time consuming and might not be possible in an emergency situation. In general, patients with uncontrolled bleeding should of course be referred for angiographic or surgical therapy.

SUMMARY AND FUTURE ASPECTS

Endoscopic hemostasis with over the scope clip is an effective technique to treat UGIB. A recent randomized controlled trial has shown superiority of over the scope clip to standard techniques for recurrent bleeding. Available retrospective studies indicate high efficacy of over the scope clip also as first-line therapy for patients at high-risk lesions. However, randomized controlled studies are urgently needed to compare over the scope clip as first-line therapy with the current standard. These studies should also clarify which subgroup of patients really benefit from over the scope clip treatment. Furthermore, factors associated with over the scope clip failure should be investigated. Finally, in the face of increasing expenses for health care, cost-effectiveness analyses are required.

SUPPLEMENTARY DATA

Supplementary data related to this article can be found online at https://doi.org/10.1016/j.giec.2019.08.001.

REFERENCES

1. Laine L, Jensen D. Management of patients with ulcer bleeding. Am J Gastroenterol 2012;107(3):345–60.
2. Lau JYW, Barkun A, Fan D, et al. Challenges in the management of acute peptic ulcer bleeding. Lancet 2013;381(9882):2033–43.
3. Camus M, Jensen DM, Kovacs TO, et al. Independent risk factors of 30-day outcomes in 1264 patients with peptic ulcer bleeding in the USA: large ulcers do worse. Aliment Pharmacol Ther 2016;43(10):1080–9.
4. Gralnek IM, Dumonceau J-M, Kuipers EJ, et al. Diagnosis and management of nonvariceal upper gastrointestinal hemorrhage: European Society of Gastrointestinal Endoscopy (ESGE) Guideline. Endoscopy 2015;47(10):a1–46.
5. Lau JY, Sung JJ, Lam YH, et al. Endoscopic retreatment compared with surgery in patients with recurrent bleeding after initial endoscopic control of bleeding ulcers. N Engl J Med 1999;340(10):751–6.
6. Nykanen T, Peltola E, Kylanpaa L, et al. Bleeding gastric and duodenal ulcers: case-control study comparing angioembolization and surgery. Scand J Gastroenterol 2017;52(5):523–30.

7. Honegger C, Valli PV, Wiegand N, et al. Establishment of Over-The-Scope-Clips (over-the-scope-clip(R)) in daily endoscopic routine. United Eur Gastroenterol J 2017;5(2):247–54.

8. Mönkemüller K, Peter S, Toshniwal J, et al. Multipurpose use of the "bear claw" (over-the-scope-clip system) to treat endoluminal gastrointestinal disorders. Dig Endosc 2014;26(3):350–7.

9. Kobara H, Mori H, Fujihara S, et al. Outcomes of gastrointestinal defect closure with an over-the-scope clip system in a multicenter experience: an analysis of a successful suction method. World J Gastroenterol 2017;23(9):1645–56.

10. Asokkumar R, Soetikno R, Sanchez-Yague A, et al. Use of over-the-scope-clip (over-the-scope clip) improves outcomes of high-risk adverse outcome (HR-AO) non-variceal upper gastrointestinal bleeding (NVUGIB). Endosc Int Open 2018;6(7):E789–96.

11. Wedi E, von Renteln D, Gonzalez S, et al. Use of the over-the-scope-clip (over-the-scope clip) in non-variceal upper gastrointestinal bleeding in patients with severe cardiovascular comorbidities: a retrospective study. Endosc Int Open 2017; 5(9):E875–82.

12. Schmidt A, Golder S, Goetz M, et al. Over-the-scope clips are more effective than standard endoscopic therapy for patients with recurrent bleeding of peptic ulcers. Gastroenterology 2018;155(3):674–86.e6.

13. Kirschniak A, Subotova N, Zieker D, et al. The Over-The-Scope Clip (over-the-scope clip) for the treatment of gastrointestinal bleeding, perforations, and fistulas. Surg Endosc 2011;25(9):2901–5.

14. Manta R, Galloro G, Mangiavillano B, et al. Over-the-scope clip (over-the-scope clip) represents an effective endoscopic treatment for acute GI bleeding after failure of conventional techniques. Surg Endosc 2013;27(9):3162–4.

15. Manno M, Mangiafico S, Caruso A, et al. First-line endoscopic treatment with over-the-scope clip in patients with high-risk non-variceal upper gastrointestinal bleeding: preliminary experience in 40 cases. Surg Endosc Other Interv Tech 2016;30(5):2026–9.

16. Wedi E, Gonzalez S, Menke D, et al. One hundred and one over-the-scope-clip applications for severe gastrointestinal bleeding, leaks and fistulas. World J Gastroenterol 2016;22(5):1844–53.

17. Richter-Schrag H-J, Glatz T, Walker C, et al. First-line endoscopic treatment with over-the-scope clips significantly improves the primary failure and rebleeding rates in high-risk gastrointestinal bleeding: a single-center experience with 100 cases. World J Gastroenterol 2016;22(41):9162–71.

18. Lamberts R, Koch A, Binner C, et al. Use of over-the-scope clips (over-the-scope clip) for hemostasis in gastrointestinal bleeding in patients under antithrombotic therapy. Endosc Int Open 2017;5(5):E324–30.

19. Wedi E, Fischer A, Hochberger J, et al. Multicenter evaluation of first-line endoscopic treatment with the over-the-scope clip in acute non-variceal upper gastrointestinal bleeding and comparison with the Rockall cohort: the FLETRock study. Surg Endosc 2018;32(1):307–14.

20. Brandler J, Baruah A, Zeb M, et al. Efficacy of over-the-scope clips in management of high-risk gastrointestinal bleeding. Clin Gastroenterol Hepatol 2018; 16(5):690–6.e1.

21. Manta R, Mangiafico S, Zullo A, et al. First-line endoscopic treatment with over-the-scope clips in patients with either upper or lower gastrointestinal bleeding: a multicenter study. Endosc Int Open 2018;6(11):E1317–21.

22. Johnston JH, Jensen DM, Auth D. Experimental comparison of endoscopic yttrium-aluminum-garnet laser, electrosurgery, and heater probe for canine gut arterial coagulation. Importance of compression and avoidance of erosion. Gastroenterology 1987;92(5 Pt 1):1101–8.
23. Chan SM, Lau JY. Can we now recommend over-the-scope clip as first-line therapy in case of non-variceal upper gastrointestinal bleeding? Endosc Int Open 2017;5(9):E883–5.
24. Naegel A, Bolz J, Zopf Y, et al. Hemodynamic efficacy of the over-the-scope clip in an established porcine cadaveric model for spurting bleeding. Gastrointest Endosc 2012;75(1):152–9.
25. Skinner M, Gutierrez JP, Neumann H, et al. Over-the-scope-clip is an effective rescue therapy for severe acute upper gastrointestinal bleeding. Endosc Int Open 2014;79(5):E37–40.
26. Schmidt A, Riecken B, Damm M, et al. Endoscopic removal of over-the-scope clips using a novel cutting device: a retrospective case series. Endoscopy 2014;46(9):762–6.
27. Bauder M, Meier B, Caca K, et al. Endoscopic removal of over-the-scope clips: clinical experience with a bipolar cutting device. United Eur Gastroenterol J 2017. https://doi.org/10.1177/2050640616671846.

Use of the Endoscopic Clipping Over the Scope Technique to Treat Acute Severe Lower Gastrointestinal Bleeding in the Colon and Anal Transition Zone

Tonya Kaltenbach, MD, MS[a,b,c,*],
Ravishankar Asokkumar, MBBS, MD, MRCP[d], Jennifer M. Kolb, MD[e],
Carmel Malvar, BA[a,b],
Roy Soetikno, MD, MS (Health Services Research), MS (Management)[c]

KEYWORDS

- Lower gastrointestinal bleeding • Endoscopic hemostasis • Endoscopic therapy
- Endoscopic clipping • Over the scope clip • Colonoscopy • Diverticular bleeding
- Anal transition zone

KEY POINTS

- Diverticular bleeding is the most common cause of acute severe lower gastrointestinal bleeding.
- Both endoscopic clipping and band ligation have been found to be safe, with extremely rare documented perforation events when used for bleeding colonic diverticula, although the endoscopic management can be technically difficult.
- There are 2 types of endoscopic clips: through the scope (TTS) and over the scope (OTS). The technique to use each clip is referred to as endoscopic clipping (C-TTS) and endoscopic clipping OTS (C-OTS).

Continued

Disclosure: Dr T. Kaltenbach is a consultant for Olympus America and Aries Pharmaceuticals, and Dr R. Soetikno is a consultant for Olympus America. Dr R. Asokkumar, Dr J.M. Kolb, and Ms C. Malvar have nothing to disclose.
[a] Section of Gastroenterology, San Francisco Veterans Affairs Medical Center, San Francisco, CA, USA; [b] Division of Gastroenterology and Hepatology, University of California, San Francisco, CA, USA; [c] Advanced Gastrointestinal Endoscopy, Mountain View, CA, USA; [d] Department of Gastroenterology and Hepatology, Singapore General Hospital, Singapore; [e] Division of Gastroenterology, University of Colorado, Aurora, CO, USA
* Corresponding author. Section of Gastroenterology, San Francisco Veterans Affairs Medical Center, San Francisco, CA.
E-mail address: endoresection@me.com

Gastrointest Endoscopy Clin N Am 30 (2020) 13–23
https://doi.org/10.1016/j.giec.2019.09.001
1052-5157/20/© 2019 Elsevier Inc. All rights reserved.

giendo.theclinics.com

Continued

- The use of the C-OTS technique has the potential to improve current treatments for diverticular bleeding. In contrast with TTS clips and band ligators, the Ovesco (Ovesco Endoscopy AG, Tubingen, Germany) clips have a much larger cap to improve visualization, capture a larger area of tissue, and have the ability to exert greater compressive force.
- Both the currently available devices for C-OTS, the Ovesco and the Padlock (US Endoscopy, Mentor, OH), are US Food and Drug Administration 510(k) cleared for the treatment of diverticular bleeding.

DEFINITIONS

This article uses the following definitions:

- Lower gastrointestinal bleeding (LGIB) refers to bleeding originating between the ileocecal valve and the anus.
- Anal transition zone (ATZ) is defined as the area interposed between the uninterrupted colorectal-type mucosa above and the uninterrupted squamous epithelium below. It starts at the dentate line and extends proximally 2 cm.
- Acute severe LGIB refers to patients with on-going bright red blood per rectum, hemodynamic instability, syncope, history of aspirin or anticoagulant use, or 2 or more comorbidities but with a nontender abdominal examination.
- There are 2 types of endoscopic clips: through the scope (TTS) and over the scope (OTS). The technique to use each clip is referred to endoscopic clipping TTS (C-TTS) and endoscopic clipping OTS (C-OTS).

INTRODUCTION

LGIB is a common cause of hospitalization in the United States.[1,2] However, the management of patients with acute severe LGIB is still evolving because data have been sparse.[3–5] Perhaps one of the reasons for the paucity of literature is that endoscopic treatment of acute severe LGIB can be technically difficult. Although diverticular bleeding is the most common cause of acute severe LGIB, isolating the bleeding diverticulum among the presence of numerous other diverticula, and, moreover, identifying and treating the bleeding site, may not be easy. At the dome, the diverticulum may not have a large enough opening to permit direct clipping. The translucent distal attachment cap can be useful in order to invert the diverticulum, expose the stigmata, and facilitate clipping.[4] Alternatively, endoscopic band ligation can be used to suction and invert the diverticulum and then place a band around it to provide hemostasis.[5] However, the use of caps, whether distal attachment or banding caps, can limit visualization because their smaller diameter causes a tunnel-like vision.

The use of the endoscopic C-OTS technique has the potential to improve current treatments for diverticular bleeding. In contrast with TTS clips and band ligators, the Ovesco clips have a much larger cap to improve visualization, capture a larger area of tissue, and have the ability to exert greater compressive force. This article summarizes our experience and the current literature on the use of the C-OTS technique to treat LGIB, specifically for colonic diverticular bleeding.

DIVERTICULAR BLEEDING
Diagnosis

The most common cause of acute severe LGIB is diverticular bleeding.[2] Although it is self-limiting for most patients, in select cases, diverticular bleeding can be massive and thus endoscopy may be a critical component of its management. The bleeding vessel, a branch of the submucosal plexus of vessels supplying the diverticulum, originates from a sizable submucosal artery. This vessel courses through the wall, dome, and neck of the diverticulum and bleeding can occur anywhere that the vessel passes through. Thus, the bleeding site can be easy or difficult to identify depending whether it is on the neck or the dome of the diverticula, respectively. Use of the distal attachment cap, placed in the long position, facilitates the detection of the bleeding vessel. Each diverticulum is investigated by inverting it with gentle suction into the cap, washing it with the water jet, and examining it closely to identify bleeding stigmata.

Treatment

Observation alone after the diagnosis of a bleeding diverticulum is associated with a high risk of rebleeding: 67% when the vessel is actively bleeding and 43% when it has an adherent clot.[3] Coaptive coagulation using a bipolar probe has been used when the bleeding site was at the neck. However, because colonic diverticula lack the muscularis propria, coagulation is generally avoided because of the risk of perforation.

The use of C-TTS to treat the bleeding diverticulum has been reported extensively.[4,6–8] When the stigmata is visible at the neck of the diverticulum, the clip can be applied directly. When the stigmata is seen inside the diverticulum, clips can be deployed to clip the neck tissue or to close the diverticular os. However, in general, these techniques are not effective. Therefore, we typically clip the bleeding vessel by using the clip from within a cap method. In this method, the clip is opened inside a cap and the diverticulum is suctioned into it.

Band ligation has also been reported extensively.[9–12] With an endoscope equipped with a band ligation device, the previously identified diverticulum is suctioned and banded at its neck. Recent literature has shown promising results for the use of band ligation for diverticular bleed hemostasis: short-term rebleeding rates after band ligation range from 3.7%[9] to 15%.[11,12] Early rebleeding (within 30 days) has been reported from band dislodgement, postbanding ulcer, or from diverticula that is different from the original bleeding source.[12] A pooled analysis showed up to 99% (95% confidence interval [CI], 95%–100%) efficacy of band ligation to treat diverticular bleeding and low early rebleeding rates of up to 8% (95% CI, 3%–16%).[13] Risk factors for early rebleeding after band ligation include younger age, active bleeding during colonoscopy, and left-sided diverticula.[12] It has been shown that using band ligation for diverticular bleeding is safe, effective, and efficient when used by both experts and training endoscopists.[14]

Rationale for Seeking Other Modalities

Endoscopic C-TTS and band ligation techniques have been found to be safe, with rare documented perforation events when used for bleeding colonic diverticula.[15] However, there are potential advantages to using the C-OTS technique that may improve the safety and efficacy of treatment. For most bleeding that occurs from within the diverticulum, clips that are deployed from within a cap or band ligation are required. However, these techniques can be difficult to perform. Further, the appropriate cap with a long barrel is not readily available and clipping from within can be complex. In addition, banding may not be feasible when the bleeding diverticulum is on the right side of the colon as its trigger cord is typically made for an upper endoscope. Banding may not be possible when the diverticulum is too small or too large and visualization through a distal attachment or banding cap may be limited because of its small diameter. In addition, OTS clips tend to stay in place longer compared with TTS clips and bands.

Use of the Clipping Over the Scope Technique

We and others have used the C-OTS technique to treat colonic diverticular bleeding, although the current literature is limited to case reports and series. The experience, as we know it, has been limited to the use of Ovesco clips, although both the Ovesco and Padlock are US Food and Drug Administration 510(k) approved for the endoscopic treatment of diverticular bleeding. In 2011, Kirschniak and colleagues[16] described the successful use of OTS clips for primary hemostasis of colonic diverticular bleeding in 2 patients. Other groups have subsequently published case reports and series (ranging from 1–6 patients) on their experience using OTS clips for primary hemostasis in patients with diverticular bleeding,[17,18] for high-risk groups on anticoagulation therapy,[19–21] and for recurrent bleeding following failed primary therapy with TTS clips.[18,22,23] In the largest published series, 2 of the 6 patients treated with the C-OTS technique for diverticular bleeding experienced in-hospital rebleeding (4 days and 13 days after C-OTS) and required additional endoscopic therapy; 1 patient was retreated with a second OTS clip and an additional 3 TTS clips, and 1 patient was retreated with fibrin glue.[20]

Our Clipping Over the Scope Technique to Treat Diverticular Bleeding in the Colon

Herein, we report our experience of treating diverticular bleeding using the endoscopic C-OTS technique. Our approach is derived from our technique for endoscopic C-TTS.[1,4] After resuscitation, we prescribe rapid large-volume colonic lavage (4–6 L until clear) using polyethylene glycol (PEG). We perform the procedure 2 hours after completion of PEG using an adult colonoscope that is equipped with water jet and carbon dioxide insufflator. We perform the procedure with the patient receiving conscious sedation with midazolam and fentanyl. We equip the colonoscope with a distal attachment cap, which is positioned long, and use it to invert the diverticulum. We use gentle suction (half suction in order to avoid injury) and wash the diverticula using the water jet. After identifying the bleeding diverticulum, we mark the suspected location using a TTS clip to indicate the area for further treatment. This clip can also be used to provide guidance to the radiologist or surgeon of the target area, if endoscopic hemostasis is not achieved.

After we identify the site of the bleeding stigmata, we then proceed with therapy using the C-OTS technique. In the setting of left-sided diverticular bleeding, we typically change the colonoscope to a therapeutic upper endoscope equipped with an OTS clipping device because the upper endoscope improves flexibility and maneuverability. Otherwise, we equip a colonoscope with an OTS clipping device (medium size). The technique of endoscopic C-OTS is similar to that of endoscopic hemorrhoid band ligation. An advantage to this system is that the diverticulum can be everted, the diverticulum suctioned, and then a single clip placed that encompasses the entire diverticulum. Compared with the endoscopic C-TTS technique, in which multiple TTS clips may be needed, the endoscopic C-OTS technique requires only a single OTS clip to ligate the entire diverticulum at the base (**Fig. 1**).

Using the endoscopic C-OTS technique, we treated 7 consecutive cases of acute severe diverticular bleeding between 2014 and 2016 at the Veterans' Affairs (VA) Palo Alto Health Care System. The institutional review board at the VA Palo Alto

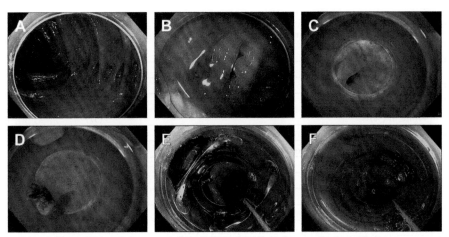

Fig. 1. Use of the endoscopic C-OTS technique to treat a colonic diverticular bleed. Following rapid bowel purge for acute severe LGIB, a patient underwent colonoscopy. (*A*) There was marked diverticulosis throughout the colon. (*B*) There was a diverticulum suspicious for bleeding stigmata features at the dome. However, the cap was too wide to invert the diverticulum. A TTS clip was placed through the scope to mark the site, and then switched to the long cap. (*C*) Using the long cap, the diverticulum was identified, and the adherent clot could be appreciated. (*D*) The diverticulum was inverted into the cap with gentle half suction to dislodge the clot and confirm the bleeding site. (*E*) The OTS clipping device was then used to advance to the bleeding diverticular site. The previously placed TTS clip was used to efficiently identify the site. (*F*) The diverticulum was then gently suctioned into the cap and the OTS clip deployed.

and Stanford University approved reporting our experiences and outcomes. Patient characteristics are reported in **Table 1**. The median age of the 7 patients was 73 years (range, 59–89 years) and all were men. The patients were American Society of Anesthesiologists (ASA) class II (5 patients) or class III (2 patients). Three patients were taking aspirin 81 mg. Otherwise, they were not on antiplatelet agents or anticoagulants. All patients were hospitalized for bleeding; 6 presented with severe bleeding, 5 of whom required intermediate intensive care unit (ICU) admission. Five had history of diverticular bleed, 2 with prior clipping, 2 with right colic embolization, and 1 with hemicolectomy. The mean plus or minus standard deviation (SD) hemoglobin decrease was 4.0 ± 2.3 g/dL (range, 0.4–6.6 g/dL). The mean ± SD time to colonoscopy was 26.9 ± 20.8 hours (range, 13–72 hours).

On endoscopy, we identified stigmata of recent hemorrhage, including active bleeding (1 patient), nonbleeding vessel (1 patient), adherent clot (6 patients), and erosion (3 patients).[4] We used a single OTS clip to achieve primary hemostasis in each patient (**Table 2**). No patient had immediate or delayed rebleeding. One patient had another bleeding episode 142 days later from a different colonic diverticulum. There were no immediate complications and no patients reported abdominal pain after C-OTS. We did not prescribe analgesic or antibiotic after the procedure. The mean ± SD number of packed red blood cells transfused was 0.71 ± 0.95 units (0–2) before colonoscopy and 0.14 ± 0.38 (0–1) after colonoscopy. The mean ± SD length of hospitalization was 3 ± 1.6 days (range, 0–5 days). The mean ± SD follow-up time for all patients was 17.6 ± 7.8 months (range, 2.1–23.3 months). The clip was still in place at 90 days on abdominal radiograph and 142 days on repeat endoscopy.

Table 1 Clinical characteristics of patients with diverticular bleeding	
Characteristic	Patients (n = 7)
Median age, y (range)	73 (59–89)
Male, n (%)	7 (100)
Race	
White, n (%)	3 (57)
African American, n (%)	4 (43)
American Society of Anesthesiologists Class	
Class II, n (%)	5 (71)
Class III, n (%)	2 (29)
Baseline Medications	
Aspirin 81 mg, n (%)	3 (43)
Plavix/warfarin/direct-acting oral anticoagulant, n (%)	0
Severe bleeding, n (%)	6 (86)
History of confirmed diverticular bleed, n (%)	5 (71)
Hemoglobin, Mean ± SD (Range)	
Baseline, g/dL	12.0 ± 2.1 (9.7–15)
Discharge, g/dL	11.0 ± 160 (9.2–13.6)
Hemoglobin decrease (g/dL)	4.0 ± 2.3 (0.4–6.6)
pRBC Transfusion, Mean ± SD (Range)	
Before colonoscopy (Units)	0.71 ± 0.95 (0–2)
Postcolonoscopy (Units)	0.14 ± 0.38 (0–1)
Colonoscopy Sedation, Mean ± SD (Range)	
Midazolam (mg)	3 ± 1.5 (1–5)
Fentanyl (µg)	96.4 ± 46.6 (25–150)
Time to colonoscopy, mean ± SD (range), h	26.9 ± 20.8 (13–72)
Instrument Used	
Upper endoscope	3 (43)
Adult colonoscope	6 (86)
Location of Bleeding in Colon	
Ascending, n (%)	3 (43)
Descending, n (%)	2 (28.5)
Sigmoid, n (%)	2 (28.5)
Stigmata of Bleeding	
Active bleeding, n (%)	1 (14)
Nonbleeding vessel, n (%)	1 (17)
Adherent clot, n (%)	6 (86)
Erosion, n (%)	3 (43)

Abbreviations: pRBC, packed red blood cells; SD, standard deviation.

POSTPOLYPECTOMY BLEEDING

After endoscopic resection of colorectal lesions, clipping may be performed in order to prevent or treat bleeding. For bleeding prophylaxis, meta-analyses have shown no significant difference for defect closure after endoscopic mucosal resection (EMR) or endoscopic submucosal dissection (ESD) for colon and rectal lesions using TTS clips

Table 2
Clinical outcomes of the 7 patients treated with the endoscopic clipping over the scope technique

Outcome (n = 7)	Patients (n = 7)
OTS clips per patient (n)	1
Primary hemostasis, n (%)	7 (100)
Rebleeding rate (n)	
Early (<30 d), n	0
Late (>30 d), n (%)	0
Follow-up, mo (range)	17.6 ± 7.8 (2.1–23.3)
Length of hospitalization, mean ± SD (range), d	3 ± 1.6 (0–5)
Patients in iICU, n (%)	5 (71%)
Complications	0

Abbreviation: iICU, intermediate ICU.

compared with no closure.[24,25] However, the studies were heterogeneous in polyp characteristics, with most polyps studied measuring less than 20 mm in diameter. Thus, the final analysis of the potential benefits of clipping after colorectal endoscopic resection is still to be determined. Notably, 2 recent large, multicenter, randomized studies have suggested a role for prophylactic clipping of large ($\geq$20 mm) postpolypectomy defects. A US study showed defect closure using TTS clips after EMR of large ($\geq$20 mm) nonpedunculated colon lesions to reduce the rate of delayed bleeding (3.5% in clip group vs 7.1% in no-clip group). Notably, the observed benefit was limited to right-sided lesions.[26] Similarly, in a Spanish trial of 235 patients with large ($\geq$20 mm) nonpedunculated colon lesions undergoing EMR, clip closure of mucosal defects was shown to reduce delayed bleeding (5% in the C-TTS group vs 12.1% in the no C-TTS group; absolute risk difference reduction of 7% in the C-TTS group; 95% CI, -14.7% to 0.3%).[27] Importantly, the protective effect of clipping depended on achievement of complete defect closure, which was achieved in only 68 cases (57%). The remaining cases had technical challenges, with partial closure in 33 cases (28%) and failed closure in 18 cases (15%). Considering such technical challenges, some investigators have studied the use of OTS clips in order to capture a larger size area and deeper tissue depth.

Use of Clipping Over the Scope Technique for the Prevention and Treatment of Postpolypectomy Bleeding

There are limited data available describing the use of the endoscopic C-OTS technique to prevent and treat bleeding after endoscopic resection in the colon.[1,21,22,28,29] Fujihara and colleagues[29] reported their experience using the endoscopic C-OTS technique for prophylactic closure of post-ESD defects. The group applied OTS clips in 9 patients who had undergone ESD of large colon lesions when the defect was determined to be too large to be closed with conventional TTS clips (resected specimen diameter: median 32 mm, range 20–55 mm) or the location was challenging, such as the hepatic flexure. No patient had bleeding postprocedure. For the treatment of delayed bleeding following endoscopic resection of colon lesions, Manta and colleagues[18] reported successful hemostasis using the endoscopic C-OTS technique in 6 cases of post-EMR (n = 5) and post-ESD (n = 1) bleeding that were refractory to conventional endoscopic therapies.

ANAL TRANSITIONAL ZONE BLEEDING

The ATZ is an area in the anal canal between the squamous epithelium of the anoderm and dentate line below and the uninterrupted rectal columnar epithelium above. The ATZ extends for a variable length (typically 1–2 cm) and its distinction from the adjacent squamous epithelium can sometimes be difficult. Unlike the squamous epithelium, the transitional lining of the ATZ is insensitive to pain. The area receives its blood supply from the superior and middle rectal artery. Bleeding occurring from this area is often poorly visualized, overlooked, or confused for hemorrhoid bleeding.

The common causes of bleeding from this area include hemorrhoids (before and after treatment), stercoral ulcers, anal fissures, and Dieulafoy lesions.[30] The data on endoscopic treatment of bleeding from the ATZ are sparse, with reported rebleeding rates as high as 48%.[30]

Our Approach for Clipping Over the Scope to Treat Bleeding in the Anal Transitional Zone

We perform endoscopic hemostasis only after cleansing the bowel with a rapid large-volume bowel purge. This purge is essential for the accurate localization of bleeding vessels and precise placement of OTS clips. We perform procedures under conscious sedation so that the patients can provide feedback as needed throughout the procedure. After identification of the bleeding site, we switch to a therapeutic upper endoscope that is equipped with a small or medium-sized OTS clipping device. The upper endoscope provides more maneuverability and allows closer access to the ATZ. We approach the lesion either in the anteflex or retroflex view. The cornerstone

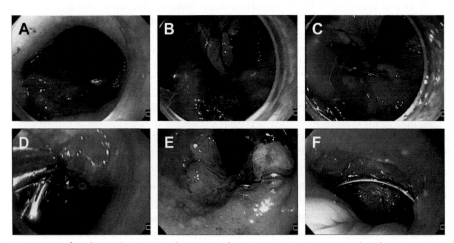

Fig. 2. Use of endoscopic C-OTS technique in the ATZ. A patient presented with acute severe LGIB 1 day following surgical hemorrhoidectomy. (*A*) There was copious fresh blood and clots visible at the anus in the distal rectum. (*B*) After suctioning and irrigation, retroflexion in the rectum showed a posthemorrhoidectomy ulcer, and (*C*) with extensive washing there was persistent and diffuse active bleeding on the distal side of the ulcer near the dentate line. (*D*) Two clips were placed using the endoscopic C-TTS technique. The area was friable and fibrosed from the hemorrhoidectomy. The bleeding continued. The scope was then mounted with the OTS clipping device to be able to clip a large surface area and suction the targeted fibrosed and friable tissue into the large cap before deployment. Hemostasis was achieved using endoscopic C-OTS technique close to the dentate line, as seen in (*E*) retroflexed and (*F*) anteflexed views.

for successful clipping is to capture the bleeding vessel without involving the squamous mucosa (**Fig. 2**). We position the cap of the OTS clip so that the bleeding lesion is captured within, but exercise special care to avoid the dentate line when suctioning the tissue into the cap. We confirm that the patient is not in pain when the mucosa is being suctioned and deploy the clip after verification. We use OTS clip accessories, such as the anchor, only when the bleeding lesion is less pliable and fibrotic.

In our prior report, we used the C-OTS technique to treat 5 patients who presented with acute severe bleeding from the ATZ caused by surgical hemorrhoidectomy (n = 2), endoscopic band ligation (n = 1), digital stimulation trauma (n = 1), and a Dieulafoy lesion (n = 1). We used a single OTS clip to achieve primary hemostasis in each patient. We successfully deployed the OTS clip in the anteflexed (n = 3) and retroflexed (n = 2) positions. None of the patients experienced immediate or delayed rebleeding and there was no recurrent bleeding at the 14-month follow-up.[31]

SUMMARY

OTS clips have been used to treat a variety of causes of acute severe LGIB, including diverticular bleeding, postpolypectomy bleeding, and ATZ bleeding, although the data are limited. Used for these indications, OTS clips may offer additional efficacy to that given by the TTS clips or band ligation devices.

ACKNOWLEDGMENTS

Presented in part at the American Society for Gastrointestinal Endoscopy Video Forum at Digestive Disease Week 2016.

REFERENCES

1. Soetikno R, Ishii N, Kolb JM, et al. The role of endoscopic hemostasis therapy in acute lower gastrointestinal hemorrhage. Gastrointest Endosc Clin N Am 2018; 28:391–408.
2. Hreinsson J, Gumundsson S, Kalaitzakis E, et al. Lower gastrointestinal bleeding: incidence, etiology, and outcomes in a population-based setting. Eur J Gastroenterol Hepatol 2013;25:37–43.
3. Jensen DM, Machicado GA, Jutabha R, et al. Urgent colonoscopy for the diagnosis and treatment of severe diverticular hemorrhage. N Engl J Med 2000; 342:78–82.
4. Kaltenbach T, Watson R, Shah J, et al. Colonoscopy with clipping is useful in the diagnosis and treatment of diverticular bleeding. Clin Gastroenterol Hepatol 2012;10:131–7.
5. Ishii N, Setoyama T, Deshpande G, et al. Endoscopic band ligation for colonic diverticular hemorrhage. Gastrointest Endosc 2012;75:382–7.
6. Yen EF, Ladabaum U, Muthusamy VR, et al. Colonoscopic treatment of acute diverticular hemorrhage using endoclips. Dig Dis Sci 2008;53:2480–5.
7. Simpson PW, Nguyen MH, Lim JK, et al. Use of endoclips in the treatment of massive colonic diverticular bleeding. Gastrointest Endosc 2004;59:433–7.
8. Kato M, Jung Y, Gromski MA, et al. Prospective, randomized comparison of 3 different hemoclips for the treatment of acute upper GI hemorrhage in an established experimental setting. Gastrointest Endosc 2012;75:3–10.
9. Shibata S, Shigeno T, Fujimori K, et al. Colonic diverticular hemorrhage: the hood method for detecting responsible diverticula and endoscopic band ligation for hemostasis. Endoscopy 2014;46:66–9.

10. Nakano K, Ishii N, Ikeya T, et al. Comparison of long-term outcomes between endoscopic band ligation and endoscopic clipping for colonic diverticular hemorrhage. Endosc Int Open 2015;3:E529–33.

11. Setoyama T, Ishii N, Fujita Y. Endoscopic band ligation (EBL) is superior to endoscopic clipping for the treatment of colonic diverticular hemorrhage. Surg Endosc 2011;25:3574–8.

12. Ikeya T, Ishii N, Nakano K, et al. Risk factors for early rebleeding after endoscopic band ligation for colonic diverticular hemorrhage. Endosc Int Open 2015;3:E523–8.

13. Ishii N, Omata F, Nagata N, et al. Effectiveness of endoscopic treatments for colonic diverticular bleeding. Gastrointest Endosc 2018;87:58–66.

14. Shimamura Y, Ishii N, Omata F, et al. Endoscopic band ligation for colonic diverticular bleeding: possibility of standardization. Endosc Int Open 2016;4:E233–7.

15. Sato Y, Yasuda H, Fukuoka A, et al. Delayed perforation after endoscopic band ligation for colonic diverticular hemorrhage. Clin J Gastroenterol 2019. https://doi.org/10.1007/s12328-019-01027-0.

16. Kirschniak A, Subotova N, Zieker D, et al. The Over-The-Scope Clip (OTSC) for the treatment of gastrointestinal bleeding, perforations, and fistulas. Surg Endosc 2011;25:2901–5.

17. Baron TH, Song LM, Ross A, et al. Use of an over-the-scope clipping device: multicenter retrospective results of the first U.S. experience (with videos). Gastrointest Endosc 2012;76:202–8.

18. Manta R, Mangiafico S, Zullo A, et al. First-line endoscopic treatment with over-the-scope clips in patients with either upper or lower gastrointestinal bleeding: a multicenter study. Endosc Int Open 2018;6:E1317–21.

19. Probst A, Braun G, Goelder S, et al. Endoscopic treatment of colonic diverticular bleeding using an over-the-scope clip. Endoscopy 2016;48(Suppl 1):E160.

20. Wedi E, von Renteln D, Jung C, et al. Treatment of acute colonic diverticular bleeding in high risk patients, using an over-the-scope clip: a case series. Endoscopy 2016;48:E383–5.

21. Richter-Schrag H-J, Glatz T, Walker C, et al. First-line endoscopic treatment with over-the-scope clips significantly improves the primary failure and rebleeding rates in high-risk gastrointestinal bleeding: a single-center experience with 100 cases. World J Gastroenterol 2016;22:9162–71.

22. Albert JG, Friedrich-Rust M, Woeste G, et al. Benefit of a clipping device in use in intestinal bleeding and intestinal leakage. Gastrointest Endosc 2011;74:389–97.

23. Kassab I, Dressner R, Gorcey S. Over-the-Scope Clip for control of a recurrent diverticular bleed. ACG Case Rep J 2015;3:5–6.

24. Nishizawa T, Suzuki H, Goto O, et al. Effect of prophylactic clipping in colorectal endoscopic resection: a meta-analysis of randomized controlled studies. United European Gastroenterol J 2017;5:859–67.

25. Boumitri C, Mir FA, Ashrf I, et al. Prophylactic clipping and post-polypectomy bleeding: a meta-analysis and systematic review. Ann Gastroenterol 2016;29:502–8.

26. Pohl H, Grimm IS, Moyer MT, et al. Clip closure prevents bleeding after endoscopic resection of large colon polyps in a randomized trial. Gastroenterology 2019;157:977–84.e3.

27. Albéniz E, Alvarez MA, Espinos JC, et al. Clip closure after resection of large colorectal lesions with substantial risk of bleeding. Gastroenterology 2019. https://doi.org/10.1053/j.gastro.2019.07.037.

28. Dinelli M, Omazzi B, Andreozzi P, et al. First clinical experiences with a novel endoscopic over-the-scope clip system. Endosc Int Open 2017;5:E151–6.
29. Fujihara S, Mori H, Kobara H, et al. The efficacy and safety of prophylactic closure for a large mucosal defect after colorectal endoscopic submucosal dissection. Oncol Rep 2013;30:85–90.
30. Daram SR, Lahr C, Tang S. Anorectal bleeding: etiology, evaluation, and management (with videos). Gastrointest Endosc 2012;76:406–17.
31. Soetikno R, Asokkumar R, Sim D, et al. Use of the over-the-scope clip to treat massive bleeding at the transitional zone of the anal canal: a case series. Gastrointest Endosc 2016;84:168–72.

Use of the Over the Scope Clip to Close Perforations and Fistulas

Panida Piyachaturawat, MD[a,b], Parit Mekaroonkamol, MD[a,b], Rungsun Rerknimitr, MD[a,b,*]

KEYWORDS

- Over the scope clip • Perforation • Fistula • Endoscopic closure

KEY POINTS

- The main advantage of endoscopic closure over surgical closure in perforation is its immediate applicability during endoscopy to prevent further spillage into peritoneal cavity.
- The over the scope clip can close a larger defect than the through the scope clip.
- The clinical success rate of the over the scope clip in perforation closure is better than that of fistula closure.

 Video content accompanies this article at http://www.giendo.theclinics.com.

INTRODUCTION

Traditionally, gastrointestinal (GI) tract disruptions, including perforation and fistula, are generally managed surgically. However, in a case with acute perforation, especially endoscopy related, an immediate surgical closure cannot be done because it requires a few hours of preparation and this delay may cause significant morbidity and mortality.[1,2] In recent years, endoscopic closure techniques, such as clipping, band ligatures, stenting, and suturing, have been developed with promising outcomes.[3–5] Many studies have supported that endoscopic closure is feasible and effective and can be considered as alternative to surgery.[6–9]

Disclosure Statement: This research received funding from a grant for International Research Integration: Chula Research Scholar; Ratchadaphiseksomphot Endowment Fund, Chulalongkorn University, and was supported by the Center of Excellence for Innovation and Endoscopy in Gastrointestinal Oncology, Faculty of Medicine, Chulalongkorn University.
[a] Division of Gastroenterology, Department of Medicine, Faculty of Medicine, Chulalongkorn University, King Chulalongkorn Memorial Hospital, Rama 4 Road, Patumwan, Bangkok 10330, Thailand; [b] Center of Excellence for Innovation and Endoscopy in Gastrointestinal Oncology, Chulalongkorn University, Bangkok, Thailand
* Corresponding author. Division of Gastroenterology, Department of Medicine, Faculty of Medicine, Chulalongkorn University, King Chulalongkorn Memorial Hospital, Rama 4 Road, Patumwan, Bangkok 10330, Thailand.
E-mail address: ercp@live.com

The through the scope clip (TTSC) is the most commonly used endoscopic modality for approximating GI defect.[4,9,10] However, TTSC cannot reliably close a deep defect larger than 1 cm unless combining it with special techniques.[11,12] The over the scope clip (over the scope clip) system (Ovesco Endoscopy AG, Tubingen, Germany) provides a more secure closure than the TTSC because of its ability to grasp full-thickness tissue. Since it has been approved by Conformite European (CE) certification in Europe in 2009 and by the US Food and Drug Administration in 2010,[13] the conventional indications for the over the scope clip therapy include GI perforations, fistulas, leakages, and refractory bleeding. In this review, we focus on the efficacy and clinical outcome of the over the scope clip for closure of perforations and fistulas.

THE OVER THE SCOPE CLIP SYSTEM

The over the scope clip system consists of an applicator cap with a mounted over the scope clip clip, thread, thread retriever, and a hand wheel for clip deployment. The applicator cap is mounted to the tip of a flexible endoscope. The target tissue is suctioned and/or grasped into the cap and the clip is then released by turning the hand wheel, using a similar technique as variceal band ligation or cap-assisted mucosal resection. The clip, which is made from nitinol, is a superelastic device designed for the compression and approximation of tissue in the GI tract.

The additional over the scope clip accessories—the Twin Grasper and Anchor forceps—are used for approximation of gapping edges or tissue defects, especially when indurated before the deployment of the over the scope clip (**Fig. 1**). The Twin Grasper forceps is preferred for fistula and perforation closures because it can separately pull the 2 opposite edges inside the over the scope clip cap. Practically, we recommend its use even in a case where suction alone can pull the designated tissue inside the cap to ensure that only the wall of the targeted tissue is suctioned (**Fig. 2**, Video 1), thus avoiding accidental entrapment of the nearby structure such as neighboring segment of bowel, bile duct, or ureter.

CLINICAL USE OF THE OVER THE SCOPE CLIP IN GASTROINTESTINAL DEFECTS

Over the scope clip was initially pioneered for hemostasis of complicated ulcer bleeding and iatrogenic perforations. Kirschniak and colleagues[14] first reported the clinical success of over the scope clip in 15 patients with severe bleeding and/or perforation. Since then, there have been several studies to support the use of over the scope clip in various indications.[15–18] In this review, we summarize the existing data on the use of over the scope clip for endoscopic closure of perforations and fistula.

DEFINITIONS

Technical success is defined as successful deployment of over the scope clip at the targeted site as determined endoscopically and/or radiographically. Clinical success is defined as the resolution of GI defects treated by the over the scope clip during a minimum 2-week follow-up as evidenced by clinical, endoscopic and/or abdominal imaging.

Perforation

In recent years, many interventional endoscopic procedures such as endoscopic submucosal dissection, per-oral endoscopic myotomy, endoscopic full-thickness resection, and endoscopic ultrasound-guided biliary and pancreatic drainage have become new frontiers in minimally-invasive management of various GI diseases. Although such

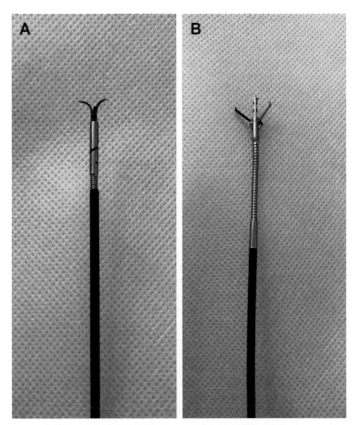

Fig. 1. The over the scope clip applicators. Anchor forceps (*A*) used for better approximation of an indurated tissue. Twin Grasper forceps (*B*) used for pulling the edges of lesion especially the large defect. (*Courtesy of* Ovesco Endoscopy AG, Tubingen, Germany.)

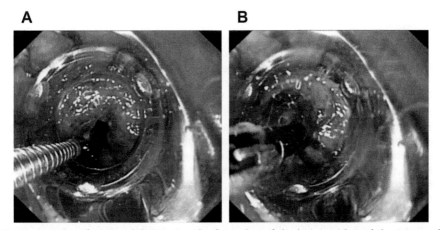

Fig. 2. Rectal perforation. (*A*) Grasping the first edge of the lesion with 1 of the 2 jaws of Twin Grasper forceps. (*B*) Grasping the opposite edge with the second jaw and retracted both edges into the cap (see Video 1). (*Courtesy of* Ovesco Endoscopy AG, Tubingen, Germany.)

advanced procedures are becoming more available, they also increase the risk of iatrogenic perforation.[19–21]

The incidence of iatrogenic endoscopic perforations is reported between as being 0.01% and 0.60% for diagnostic and 0.6% and 5.5% for therapeutic endoscopies.[1,11,22] Although the incidence is considerably low, this serious adverse event is associated with significant morbidity and mortality.

Early detection is the key factor for the optimal outcome in the management of perforation because it allows a prompt closure to reduce the risk of further spillage of GI content.

Practically, TTSC is the most commonly used device. The most suitable perforation diameter for the TTSC perforation closure are those smaller than 1 cm or linear perforation.[9] The TTSC closure on nonlinear perforations larger than 1 cm can be challenging and may require addition accessories or different technique, such as endoloop or banding.[23,24] Therefore, an easier to use system, such as over the scope clip, is generally preferred for an immediate closure in such challenging cases. Technically, the over the scope clip could be used to the defective area in the location as deep as the standard end-viewing endoscope (a diameter of 8.5–14.0 mm) can reach.

Based on our systematic review using the search terms "perforation," "full thickness defect," and "over the scope clip" in Pubmed and the Cochrane Central Register of Controlled Trials up until February 2019, there were 19 studies published in English language. A total of 319 patients were included. The overall technical success rate (TSR) and clinical success rate (CSR) were 91% and 84%, respectively (**Table 1**).

Kirschniak and colleagues[15] first reported a 100% TSR and CSR for closure of 11 perforations, 7 in the upper and 4 in the lower GI tract. Haito-Chavez and colleagues[17] reported a CSR of 90% in 48 perforations (21% esophagus, 27% stomach, 19% duodenum, 17% colon, and 9% rectum) with a median diameter of 7 mm (range, 4–12 mm).

Honegger and colleagues[18] reported the largest study of 72 perforations and achieved 90% endoscopic closure using over the scope clip with the highest TSR in colon (96%) and duodenum (90%), although it was lowest in esophagus (77%) and small bowel (78%). The difficulty was explained by the tangential endoscopic view in a relatively small diameter esophageal lumen. The lower success rate in small bowel closure was blamed on its very active peristaltic movement and its unreachable depth.

Voermans and colleagues[25] demonstrated a 92% TSR in 36 patients with acute perforations (5 esophageal, 6 gastric, 12 duodenal, and 13 colonic perforations). All failed cases were patients with duodenal perforation owing to the inability to maneuver the endoscope in a proper position to place the over the scope clip.

A relatively lower CSR of 64.7% and 57.0% were reported by Hagel and colleagues[26] and Wedi and colleagues,[27] respectively. Failed cases were attributed to the lesions with necrotic, severely inflamed ischemic, retracted or fixed margins, perforation size larger than 20 mm, perforation that existed more than 72 hours, and perforation located at the proximal to mid esophagus.

Mangiavillano and colleagues[28] categorized perforations based on their shape, namely, round and oval. They found that in, contrast with the oval configuration, round defects were more difficult to be adequately suctioned into the over the scope clip cap. They required Twin Grasper forceps to approximate the edges before closure. However, the tissue condition and size of the defects were not reported, which could have also been confounding factors, rather than the shape of the defect alone.

Kobara and colleagues[29] in a series of 28 patients treated by over the scope clip demonstrated that closure of the defect was possible in perforation up to 30 mm.

Table 1					
Clinical outcomes of the over the scope clip system for perforation closure					
Author (Reference) and Year	Country	Patients (n)	Size (mm)	CSR (%)	Complications (%)
Parodi et al,[55] 2010	Italy	4	5–20	75	n/a
Kirsckniak et al,[15] 2011	Germany	11	n/a	100	n/a
Albert et al,[43] 2011	Germany	2	n/a	100	n/a
Voermans et al,[25] 2012	The Netherlands	36	n/a	89	2.8
Baron et al,[48] 2012	USA	5	n/a	80	n/a
Hagel et al[26] 2012	Germany	17	6–40	65	5.9
Jayaraman et al,[16] 2013	USA	6	5–25	75	n/a
Haito-Chavez et al,[17] 2014	International	48	4–12	90	0
Angsuwatcharakon et al,[56] 2016	Thailand	6	10–14	84	0
Mizrahi et al,[46] 2016	USA	4	n/a	75	0
Donatelli et al,[57] 2016	France	15	10–20	100	0
Wedi et al,[27] 2016	International	7	n/a	57	2
Mangiavillano et al,[28] 2016	Italy	20	3–18	90	0
Raithel et al,[52] 2017	Germany	22	n/a	73	8.8
Goenka et al,[58] 2017	India	3	n/a	100	n/a
Kobara et al,[29] 2017	Japan	28	3–50	93	n/a
Honegger et al,[18] 2017	Switzerland	72	n/a	86	n/a
Khater et al,[59] 2017	France	11	10–20	82	9.1
Lee et al,[47] 2018	Korea	2	10–30	100	n/a
Total % (n)		319		84 (267/319)	1.8 6/319

Abbreviation: n/a, not applicable.

Twin Grasper forceps was claimed as very useful in 72% of patients whose defect was larger than 10 mm.

From our experience, endoscopic retrograde cholangiopancreatography and endoscopic ultrasound-related duodenal perforation are very challenging. Owing to the typical C-loop anatomy of duodenum, it may be difficult to place the over the scope clip in certain angles.

If the perforation is scope induced, it usually locates at 2 locations. One is on the antimesenteric side of duodenal bulb from postpyloric duodenoscope intubation and the other is on the antimesenteric side of the second part of duodenum, usually from a stone extraction maneuver. The over the scope clip closure for these 2 locations is quite possible if the diameter of the perforation is less than 3 cm (**Figs. 3** and **4**, Video 2). However, if the perforation develops at the ampullary site and the mechanism is from cauterization after sphincterotomy or ampullectomy, the closure

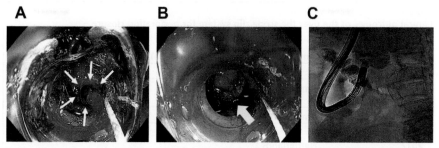

Fig. 3. Iatrogenic perforation caused by echoendoscope developed at duodenal bulb. (*A*) The perforation site was targeted with over the scope clip cap (the *white arrow* shows the edge of defect). (*B*) After over the scope clip deployment (*yellow arrow*, over the scope clip). (*C*) Contrast was instilled to perforation site to confirm a completer closure. (*Courtesy of* Ovesco Endoscopy AG, Tubingen, Germany.)

is technically demanding because of the awkward endoscopic position and the risk of over the scope clip entrapping biliary and pancreatic orifices. In this situation, we recommend placing both biliary and pancreatic stents first before replacing a duodenoscope with an end-viewing gastroscope. The over the scope clip cap can be used to push the 2 stents aside from the deployment location (**Fig. 5**, Video 3). Regarding the location and diameter of perforation, we have summarized our recommended endoscopic closure techniques in **Table 2**.

CONTRAINDICATIONS FOR OVER THE SCOPE CLIP CLOSURE IN PERFORATION

The use of over the scope clip should be with caution when the perforation is detected after 24 hours[4,25,26] owing to concern for peritoneal contamination and the poor tissue healing from delayed closure. Colonic perforation in the setting of poor bowel preparation is also not a good indication for over the scope clip closure because the risk of peritoneal contamination is very high, even with early detection. From our experience, a large defect that fails closure attempts using 2 over the scope clip should be directed to surgery.

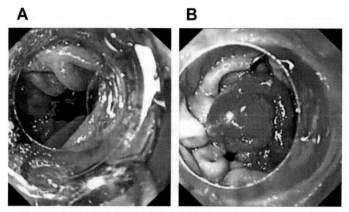

Fig. 4. Duodenal perforation during stone extraction developed at the antimesenteric site of the second part of duodenum; see Video 2. (*A*) Before over the scope clip deployment. (*B*) After over the scope clip deployment. (*Courtesy of* Ovesco Endoscopy AG, Tubingen, Germany.)

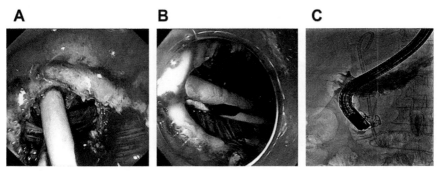

Fig. 5. (*A*) Duodenoscopic view of a postampullectomy related perforation with biliary and pancreatic stents already placed. (*B*) A view from an end-viewing endoscope demonstrated a very large defect. (*C*) Enterogram confirmed a complete closure (see Video 3).

Fistula

A fistula is an abnormal communication between the 2 organs via an epithelialized tract. Unlike perforation, fistula consists of fibrotic tissue that can be difficult for endoscopic manipulation. Common GI tract fistulas are (1) an airway-connected fistula, that is, tracheoesophageal, bronchoesophageal, or bronchogastric fistula, which are mostly secondary to malignant conditions or prolonged mechanical ventilation. Closure of this fistula is mandatory because of the risk for recurrent aspiration pneumonia (**Fig. 6**);[30,31] (2) Gastroduodenal fistula that usually develops after surgery;[32,33] (3) Gastrocutaneous fistula that usually occurs after the removal of percutaneous endoscopic gastrostomy tube. Although many of these fistulas spontaneously closed after a short period of time, some might require an intervention;[34,35] (4) Colonic fistulas often communicate with the bladder, vagina, or skin. The main etiologies are diverticular disease, Crohn's disease, invading tumor, radiation therapy, or trauma.[36,37]

Current endoscopic treatments for GI fistula include the placement of covered metal stents, fibrin glue injection, and placement of the TTSC. Unfortunately, these approaches have several limitations.[38,39] The placement of covered metal stents

Table 2
Recommended closure techniques according to the location and diameter of perforations

Location	Size of Perforation (mm)		
	<10	≥10 and <30	≥30
Esophagus	TTSC	over the scope clip	Esophageal FCSEMS or 2 over the scope clips or surgery
Stomach	TTSC	over the scope clip	Two over the scope clips or surgery
Duodenal wall	TTSC	over the scope clip	Two over the scope clips or surgery
Sphincterotomy-related	Standard biliary FCSEMS or TTSC	Large FCSEMS	n/a
Colon and rectum (Good bowel preparation)	TTSC	over the scope clip	Two over the scope clips or surgery

Abbreviations: FCSEMS, fully-covered self-expandable metallic stent; n/a, not applicable.

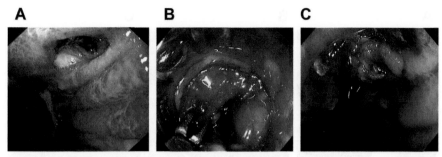

Fig. 6. (*A*) A 10-mm defect with inflammation edge detected at the lessor curvature of stomach with the opposite lumen being the left main bronchus, (*B*) By using a double-channel gastroscope, 2 rat-tooth forceps were used for grasping the 2 edges of the defect and suctioned them into the cap. (*C*) The over the scope clip was successfully deployed for a complete closure of bronchogastric fistula. (*Courtesy of* Ovesco Endoscopy AG, Tubingen, Germany.)

sometimes leads to insufficient closure, early stent migration, or stent-induced strictures.[38–40] Glue injection is only indicated for fistula smaller than 5 mm in diameter.[41,42] TTSC can only grasp superficial mucosa and is not reliably effective even for a small fistula. In contrast, the over the scope clip is considered superior because it can grasp the full thickness of the fistula edge for a closure.

Based on our systematic review using the search terms "fistula" and "over the scope clip" in Pubmed and the Cochrane Central Register of Controlled Trials up to February 2019, there are 20 studies published in English language. A total 437 patients were included and finding are summarized in **Table 3**. Although the overall TSR was 80% (range, 50%–100%), the overall CSR was only 48% (range, 25%–100%).

There were discrepancies between TSR and CSR reported in many studies.[17,18,43–47] Kirschniak and colleagues[15] reported 88% TSR (7/8) with only 38% CSR. The majority of the upper GI tract fistula in this study were percutaneous endoscopic gastrostomy related. All 3 cases of colonic fistulas failures were caused by either malignancy or inflammation from pancreatitis. They recurred between 7 to 11 days after the intervention. Mizrahi and colleagues[46] also showed a low CSR of 35% with all over the scope clip failures were in lower GI fistulae. Similarly, Haito-Chavez and colleagues[17] and Honegger and colleagues[18] reported only 43% and 29% CSR despite the high TSR of more than 80%.

The main causes of over the scope clip placement failure were the nonsuitable anatomic structure, the rigidity of lesion-surrounding tissue, and the lesion diameter exceeding the capacity of successful approach by the over the scope clip, whereas the reasons for the lower CSR remain unclear. We speculate that the poor tissue integrity and the spontaneous recanalization of the tract may have played the important roles. We also suspect that the etiologies of the fistula that preclude normal tissue healing that is inflammatory bowel disease related, radiation induced, a surgical complication, or malignancy related would have contributed to the difference in CSR. Unfortunately, data from such subgroup analyses were not available.

Albert and colleagues[43] suggested that the Twin Grasper forceps could add benefit over the technique of simple suction and they strongly advised for a large lesion (>1–2 cm), because sometimes suction alone may unintentionally trap the nearby structure. Baron and colleagues[48] also suggested the use of the anchoring

Table 3
Clinical outcomes of the over the scope clip system for fistula closure

Author (Reference) and Year	Patients (n)	Location	Size (mm)	TSR (%)	CSR (%)
Parodi et al,[55] 2010	5	Gastrocutaneous, Colocutaneous, Gastromediastinal, Colovesical, Colorectal	10–15	80	80
Kirsckniak et al,[15] 2011	8	Gastrocutaneous Esophagojejunostomy Rectovaginal Colocutaneous	n/a	88	38
Albert et al,[43] 2011	6	Gastrocutaneous Enterocutaneous Gastrojejunal	n/a	75	25
Surace et al,[49] 2011	19	Gastrocutaneous Rectovaginal	n/a	91	74
Baron et al,[48] 2012	28	n/a	n/a	n/a	68
Jayaraman et al,[16] 2013	11	n/a	5–25	84	67
Monkenuller et al,[44] 2014	6	TE fistula, gastrocutaneous	3–15	100	50
Haito-Chavez et al,[17] 2014	108	Esophagogastric, esophagopleural, tracheoesophageal, gastrocutaneous, rectum	4–10	94	43
Sulz et al,[60] 2014	11	n/a	2–20	85	64
Mercky et al,[50] 2015	30	n/a	3–20	71	53
Singhal et al,[35] 2015	10	PEG	6–20	100	90
Law et al,[45] 2015	47	n/a	n/a	89	53
Mizrahi et al,[46] 2016	17	Bronchoesophageal, Gastrocutaneous, Enterocutaneous	n/a	100	35
Donatelli et al,[57] 2016	30	Upper GI (29), lower GI (1)	10–20	50	37
Winder et al,[61] 2016	22	n/a	n/a	n/a	77
Wedi et al,[27] 2016	3	Gastrocutaneous, pseudocyst	n/a	100	100
Goenka et al,[58] 2017	3	Esophagopleural, colonopseudoscyst	n/a	67	67
Kobara et al,[29] 2017	12	Gastrocutaneous, rectovesical, gastropseudocyst, colon-GB	3–50	90	82
Honegger et al,[18] 2017	57	n/a	n/a	80	30
Lee et al,[47] 2018	4	Bronchoesophageal Gastrocolonic Colonopseudocyst	5–20	100	25
Total % (n)	437			80 (350/437)	48 (211/437)

Abbreviations: GB, gallbladder; GI, gastrointestinal; n/a, not applicable; PEG, percutaneous endoscopic gastrostomy; TE, tracheoesophageal.

device to hold the tissue in those with chronic, fibrotic ulcers, particularly in the setting of prior radiation therapy where tissue healing is compromised.

In most studies,[15,18,43,49,50] the over the scope clip system failure occurred within a median time of 2 weeks (range, 5 days to 4 weeks) after treatment. This finding probably reflects the chronicity of the lesions and it implies that simple closure of the fistulous opening may not be sufficient if the underlying etiology is not adequately controlled.

THE STEPS FOR OVER THE SCOPE CLIP CLOSURE

1. To avoid overdistension of the abdomen and not compromising respiratory mechanic of the patient, we recommend using carbon dioxide insufflation, or minimizing overinsufflation by room air if a carbon dioxide system is not available.
2. If the perforation develops in the area that may be difficult to locate such as area behind the fold or post bulbar, marking the nearby mucosa with cauterization is recommended. Because the endoscopic visualization will be compromised after mounting the over the scope clip cap.
3. Twin Grasper forceps, rather than suctioning alone, should be used when available to avoid accidental entrapment of the wall of nearby structures.
4. Twin Grasper forceps should be held tightly using the left hand (**Fig. 7**) to make sure that all parts of the forceps and the targeted edges are suctioned and well-maintained inside the over the scope clip cap before deployment.

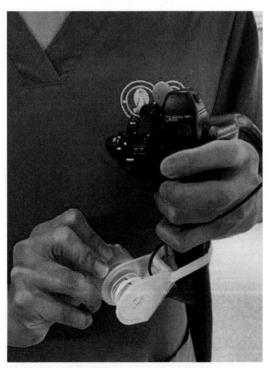

Fig. 7. Holding the Twin Grasper forceps very tight by using the left hand to control and to make sure that all the parts of the Twin Grasper and mucosa are pulled completely into the cap before deployment. (*Courtesy of* Ovesco Endoscopy AG, Tubingen, Germany.)

A   **B**   **C**

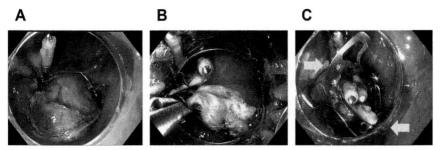

Fig. 8. (A) A 45-mm defect was seen after an endoscopic submucosal dissection of a large duodenal stromal tumor and subsequently through the scope clipping failed. (B) Using a Twin Grasper to retract the lower edge of defect into the cap. (C) Successful closure of the large defect by using 2 over the scope clips placed tandemly (*yellow arrow*). ([B, C] *Courtesy of* Ovesco Endoscopy AG, Tubingen, Germany.)

5. Closure confirmation by contrast instillation or water distension if fluoroscopy is not available is recommended to confirm sealing.
6. In a large defect wherein 1 over the scope clip placement is insufficient, a second over the scope clip can be placed beside the first one without entrapping the edge of the first over the scope clip while a small gap is allowed in between the 2 over the scope clips (**Fig. 8**).

OVER THE SCOPE CLIP–ASSOCIATED COMPLICATIONS

Over the scope clip-related complication has been reported in 1.8% of cases.[51] One case of esophageal perforation developed during an introduction of the over the scope clip-mounted endoscope and 3 cases of peritonitis have been reported.[25,52] Other complications included intraluminal stenosis, accidental entrapment of adjacent structures, minor tongue injury, and ureteric obstruction and small bowel fixation.[43,48,50,53,54] Twin Grasper forceps or the over the scope clip anchor, rather than suctioning alone, could have minimized the risk of these complications.

SUMMARY

The over the scope clip is a safe and effective device when used in a proper setting. In patients with iatrogenic perforation and fistula, prompt endoscopic closure using over the scope clip has become a promising approach. The main advantage of over the scope clip over the conventional TTSC is its ability to close large nonlinear defect of up to 3 cm. More than 1 over the scope clip may be applied tandemly for larger defects. The overall CSR of over the scope clip in perforation closure is much better than that for fistula, especially fistula with the presence of thickened or fibrotic mucosal edges, scar, active inflammation, or infiltrating malignancy.

SUPPLEMENTARY DATA

Supplementary data related to this article can be found online at https://doi.org/10.1016/j.giec.2019.08.002.

REFERENCES

1. Luning TH, Keemers-Gels ME, Barendregt WB, et al. Colonoscopic perforations: a review of 30,366 patients. Surg Endosc 2007;21(6):994–7.

2. Iqbal CW, Cullinane DC, Schiller HJ, et al. Surgical management and outcomes of 165 colonoscopic perforations from a single institution. Arch Surg 2008;143(7): 701–6 [discussion: 706–7].
3. Putcha RV, Burdick JS. Management of iatrogenic perforation. Gastroenterol Clin North Am 2003;32(4):1289–309.
4. Paspatis GA, Dumonceau JM, Barthet M, et al. Diagnosis and management of iatrogenic endoscopic perforations: European Society of Gastrointestinal Endoscopy (ESGE) Position Statement. Endoscopy 2014;46(8):693–711.
5. Singh RR, Nussbaum JS, Kumta NA. Endoscopic management of perforations, leaks and fistulas. Transl Gastroenterol Hepatol 2018;3:85.
6. Mangiavillano B, Viaggi P, Masci E. Endoscopic closure of acute iatrogenic perforations during diagnostic and therapeutic endoscopy in the gastrointestinal tract using metallic clips: a literature review. J Dig Dis 2010;11(1):12–8.
7. van Heel NC, Haringsma J, Spaander MC, et al. Short-term esophageal stenting in the management of benign perforations. Am J Gastroenterol 2010;105(7): 1515–20.
8. Heits N, Stapel L, Reichert B, et al. Endoscopic endoluminal vacuum therapy in esophageal perforation. Ann Thorac Surg 2014;97(3):1029–35.
9. Yilmaz B, Unlu O, Roach EC, et al. Endoscopic clips for the closure of acute iatrogenic perforations: where do we stand? Dig Endosc 2015;27(6):641–8.
10. Verlaan T, Voermans RP, van Berge Henegouwen MI, et al. Endoscopic closure of acute perforations of the GI tract: a systematic review of the literature. Gastrointest Endosc 2015;82(4):618–28.e5.
11. Minami S, Gotoda T, Ono H, et al. Complete endoscopic closure of gastric perforation induced by endoscopic resection of early gastric cancer using endoclips can prevent surgery (with video). Gastrointest Endosc 2006;63(4):596–601.
12. Biancari F, Saarnio J, Mennander A, et al. Outcome of patients with esophageal perforations: a multicenter study. World J Surg 2014;38(4):902–9.
13. Committee AT, Banerjee S, Barth BA, et al. Endoscopic closure devices. Gastrointest Endosc 2012;76(2):244–51.
14. Kirschniak A, Kratt T, Stuker D, et al. A new endoscopic over-the-scope clip system for treatment of lesions and bleeding in the GI tract: first clinical experiences. Gastrointest Endosc 2007;66(1):162–7.
15. Kirschniak A, Subotova N, Zieker D, et al. The Over-The-Scope Clip (over-the-scope clip) for the treatment of gastrointestinal bleeding, perforations, and fistulas. Surg Endosc 2011;25(9):2901–5.
16. Jayaraman V, Hammerle C, Lo SK, et al. Clinical application and outcomes of over the scope clip device: initial US experience in humans. Diagn Ther Endosc 2013;2013:381873.
17. Haito-Chavez Y, Law JK, Kratt T, et al. International multicenter experience with an over-the-scope clipping device for endoscopic management of GI defects (with video). Gastrointest Endosc 2014;80(4):610–22.
18. Honegger C, Valli PV, Wiegand N, et al. Establishment of Over-The-Scope-Clips (over-the-scope clip(R)) in daily endoscopic routine. United European Gastroenterol J 2017;5(2):247–54.
19. Silviera ML, Seamon MJ, Porshinsky B, et al. Complications related to endoscopic retrograde cholangiopancreatography: a comprehensive clinical review. J Gastrointest Liver Dis 2009;18(1):73–82.
20. Ojima T, Takifuji K, Nakamura M, et al. Complications of endoscopic submucosal dissection for gastric noninvasive neoplasia: an analysis of 647 lesions. Surg Laparosc Endosc Percutan Tech 2014;24(4):370–4.

21. Sato H, Inoue H, Ikeda H, et al. Clinical experience of esophageal perforation occurring with endoscopic submucosal dissection. Dis Esophagus 2014;27(7): 617–22.
22. Stapfer M, Selby RR, Stain SC, et al. Management of duodenal perforation after endoscopic retrograde cholangiopancreatography and sphincterotomy. Ann Surg 2000;232(2):191–8.
23. Katsinelos P, Chatzimavroudis G, Terzoudis S, et al. The endoloop-clips technique for closure of large iatrogenic colonic perforations. Endoscopy 2010;42(4):343 [author reply: 344].
24. Ryu JY, Park BK, Kim WS, et al. Endoscopic closure of iatrogenic colon perforation using dual-channel endoscope with an endoloop and clips: methods and feasibility data (with videos). Surg Endosc 2019;33(4):1342–8.
25. Voermans RP, Le Moine O, von Renteln D, et al. Efficacy of endoscopic closure of acute perforations of the gastrointestinal tract. Clin Gastroenterol Hepatol 2012; 10(6):603–8.
26. Hagel AF, Naegel A, Lindner AS, et al. Over-the-scope clip application yields a high rate of closure in gastrointestinal perforations and may reduce emergency surgery. J Gastrointest Surg 2012;16(11):2132–8.
27. Wedi E, Gonzalez S, Menke D, et al. One hundred and one over-the-scope-clip applications for severe gastrointestinal bleeding, leaks and fistulas. World J Gastroenterol 2016;22(5):1844–53.
28. Mangiavillano B, Caruso A, Manta R, et al. Over-the-scope clips in the treatment of gastrointestinal tract iatrogenic perforation: a multicenter retrospective study and a classification of gastrointestinal tract perforations. World J Gastrointest Surg 2016;8(4):315–20.
29. Kobara H, Mori H, Fujihara S, et al. Outcomes of gastrointestinal defect closure with an over-the-scope clip system in a multicenter experience: an analysis of a successful suction method. World J Gastroenterol 2017;23(9):1645–56.
30. Reed MF, Mathisen DJ. Tracheoesophageal fistula. Chest Surg Clin N Am 2003; 13(2):271–89.
31. Balazs A, Kupcsulik PK, Galambos Z. Esophagorespiratory fistulas of tumorous origin. Non-operative management of 264 cases in a 20-year period. Eur J Cardiothoracic Surg 2008;34(5):1103–7.
32. Falconi M, Pederzoli P. The relevance of gastrointestinal fistulae in clinical practice: a review. Gut 2001;49(Suppl 4):iv2–10.
33. Oda I, Suzuki H, Nonaka S, et al. Complications of gastric endoscopic submucosal dissection. Dig Endosc 2013;25(Suppl 1):71–8.
34. McElrath L, Pauli EM, Marks JM. Hernia formation and persistent fistula after percutaneous endoscopy gastrostomy: unusual complications of a common procedure. Am Surg 2012;78(4):E200–1.
35. Singhal S, Changela K, Culliford A, et al. Endoscopic closure of persistent gastrocutaneous fistulae, after percutaneous endoscopic gastrostomy (PEG) tube placement, using the over-the-scope-clip system. Therap Adv Gastroenterol 2015;8(4):182–8.
36. Wolfe FD. Colonic fistula: causes and management. J Int Coll Surg 1961;35: 101–4.
37. Annibali R, Pietri P. Fistulous complications of Crohn's disease. Int Surg 1992; 77(1):19–27.
38. Amrani L, Menard C, Berdah S, et al. From iatrogenic digestive perforation to complete anastomotic disunion: endoscopic stenting as a new concept of

"stent-guided regeneration and re-epithelialization". Gastrointest Endosc 2009; 69(7):1282–7.

39. Bege T, Emungania O, Vitton V, et al. An endoscopic strategy for management of anastomotic complications from bariatric surgery: a prospective study. Gastrointest Endosc 2011;73(2):238–44.

40. Pohl J, Borgulya M, Lorenz D, et al. Endoscopic closure of postoperative esophageal leaks with a novel over-the-scope clip system. Endoscopy 2010;42(9): 757–9.

41. Tsunezuka Y, Sato H, Tsukioka T, et al. A new instrument for endoscopic gluing for bronchopleural fistulae. Ann Thorac Surg 1999;68(3):1088–9.

42. Yoon JH, Lee HL, Lee OY, et al. Endoscopic treatment of recurrent congenital tracheoesophageal fistula with Histoacryl glue via the esophagus. Gastrointest Endosc 2009;69(7):1394–6.

43. Albert JG, Friedrich-Rust M, Woeste G, et al. Benefit of a clipping device in use in intestinal bleeding and intestinal leakage. Gastrointest Endosc 2011;74(2): 389–97.

44. Monkemuller K, Peter S, Toshniwal J, et al. Multipurpose use of the 'bear claw' (over-the-scope-clip system) to treat endoluminal gastrointestinal disorders. Dig Endosc 2014;26(3):350–7.

45. Law R, Wong K, Song LM, et al. Immediate technical and delayed clinical outcome of fistula closure using an over-the-scope clip device. Surg Endosc 2015;29(7):1781–6.

46. Mizrahi I, Eltawil R, Haim N, et al. The clinical utility of over-the-scope clip for the treatment of gastrointestinal defects. J Gastrointest Surg 2016;20(12):1942–9.

47. Lee HL, Cho JY, Cho JH, et al. Efficacy of the over-the-scope clip system for treatment of gastrointestinal fistulas, leaks, and perforations: a Korean multi-center study. Clin Endosc 2018;51(1):61–5.

48. Baron TH, Song LM, Ross A, et al. Use of an over-the-scope clipping device: multicenter retrospective results of the first U.S. experience (with videos). Gastrointest Endosc 2012;76(1):202–8.

49. Surace M, Mercky P, Demarquay JF, et al. Endoscopic management of GI fistulae with the over-the-scope clip system (with video). Gastrointest Endosc 2011;74(6): 1416–9.

50. Mercky P, Gonzalez JM, Aimore Bonin E, et al. Usefulness of over-the-scope clipping system for closing digestive fistulas. Dig Endosc 2015;27(1):18–24.

51. Kobara H, Mori H, Nishiyama N, et al. Over-the-scope clip system: a review of 1517 cases over 9 years. J Gastroenterol Hepatol 2019;34(1):22–30.

52. Raithel M, Albrecht H, Scheppach W, et al. Outcome, comorbidity, hospitalization and 30-day mortality after closure of acute perforations and postoperative anastomotic leaks by the over-the-scope clip (over-the-scope clip) in an unselected cohort of patients. Surg Endosc 2017;31(6):2411–25.

53. Albrecht H, Naegel A, Hagel A, et al. Over-the-scope-clipping in colonic perforation caused small-bowel fixation and pneumoperitoneum requiring surgical repair. Endoscopy 2014;46(Suppl 1 UCTN):E314–5.

54. Rahmi G, Barret M, Samaha E, et al. Ureteral obstruction after colonoscopic perforation closed with an over-the-scope clip. Gastrointest Endosc 2015;81(2): 470–1 [discussion: 471–2].

55. Parodi A, Repici A, Pedroni A, et al. Endoscopic management of GI perforations with a new over-the-scope clip device (with videos). Gastrointest Endosc 2010; 72(4):881–6.

56. Angsuwatcharakon P, Prueksapanich P, Kongkam P, et al. Efficacy of the ovesco clip for closure of endoscope related perforations. Diagn Ther Endosc 2016; 2016:9371878.
57. Donatelli G, Cereatti F, Dhumane P, et al. Closure of gastrointestinal defects with Ovesco clip: long-term results and clinical implications. Therap Adv Gastroenterol 2016;9(5):713–21.
58. Goenka MK, Rai VK, Goenka U, et al. Endoscopic management of gastrointestinal leaks and bleeding with the over-the-scope clip: a prospective study. Clin Endosc 2017;50(1):58–63.
59. Khater S, Rahmi G, Perrod G, et al. Over-the-scope clip (over-the-scope clip) reduces surgery rate in the management of iatrogenic gastrointestinal perforations. Endosc Int Open 2017;5(5):E389–94.
60. Sulz MC, Bertolini R, Frei R, et al. Multipurpose use of the over-the-scope-clip system ("Bear claw") in the gastrointestinal tract: Swiss experience in a tertiary center. World J Gastroenterol 2014;20(43):16287–92.
61. Winder JS, Kulaylat AN, Schubart JR, et al. Management of non-acute gastrointestinal defects using the over-the-scope clips (over-the-scope clips): a retrospective single-institution experience. Surg Endosc 2016;30(6):2251–8.

16.

17.

18.

19.

20.

The Use of the Over the Scope Clips Beyond Its Standard Use: A Pictorial Description

Klaus Mönkemüller, MD, PhD[a,b,c],*, Alvaro Martínez-Alcalá, MD[d], Arthur R. Schmidt, MD, PhD[e], Thomas Kratt, MD[f]

KEYWORDS

- Gastrointestinal perforations • Gastrointestinal leaks • Gastrointestinal dehiscence
- Over the scope clips • Ovesco • Endoscopic suturing devices • Bear claw

KEY POINTS

- The over the scope clips is a tissue apposition device made of Nitinol.
- Because of its tissue apposition capabilities, the over the scope clip can be used for closure of perforations and fistulae, to treat gastrointestinal bleeding and to anchor self-expanding metal stents.
- The over the scope clips is used as a single therapy or as part of a multimodal combination approach to treat complex endoluminal gastrointestinal disorders.

 Video content accompanies this article at http://www.giendo.theclinics.com.

INTRODUCTION

The over the scope clips (over the scope clips; Ovesco, Tübingen, Germany), which was also baptized as "bear claw" or "bear trap," is an endoscopic clipping device made of Nitinol designed for tissue approximation.[1–5] As such, it was originally used for the closure of fistulas and perforations.[3–6] Because of its apposition force and easy en face application, its uses have been expanded to include the therapy for bleeding lesions, resection of submucosal tumors, and esophageal stent fixation.[7–12]

---

[a] Department of Gastroenterology, Helios Frankenwaldklinik, Kronach, Germany; [b] Department of Gastroenterology, Otto-von-Guericke University, Magdeburg, Germany; [c] University of Belgrade, Belgrade, Serbia; [d] Department of Gastroenterology, Hospital Universitario Infanta Leonor, Madrid, Spain; [e] Division of Interdisciplinary Endoscopy, University of Freiburg, Germany; [f] Department of Surgery, University of Heidelberg, Heidelberg, Germany
* Corresponding author. Department of Gastroenterology, Helios Frankenwaldklinik, Kronach, Germany.
E-mail address: moenkemueller@yahoo.com

Gastrointest Endoscopy Clin N Am 30 (2020) 41–74
https://doi.org/10.1016/j.giec.2019.09.003
1052-5157/20/© 2019 Elsevier Inc. All rights reserved.

The uses of over the scope clips have expanded beyond simple closure of fistulae or perforations. Now the device is also used to treat more complex defects of the luminal gastrointestinal tract. More importantly, the over the scope clips is also used during multimodal closure of gastrointestinal wall defects.[1,6,13] At present, endoscopic prophylaxis and management of perforations associated with endoluminal lesion resection have been expanded using the over the scope clips, by using the clip to close evident or potential perforations.[13–17] Last but not least, the over the scope clips device may become a preferred device to treat bleeding ulcers located in difficult positions because of its barrel-shaped transparent cap design, which allows suctioning the bleeding lesion.[18–20] Although using the over the scope clips system is generally straightforward, it is essential that the therapeutic endoscopist has a clear understanding of the advantages and potential limitations of this device. The objectives of this atlas are to describe uses of over the scope clips beyond traditional indications, including larger defects and uses beyond routine indications. We specifically describe key technical aspects and potential limitations of these devices in the context of these challenging clinical situations.

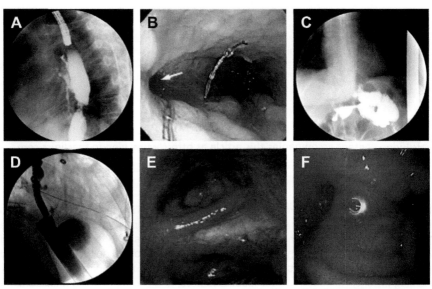

Fig. 1. Gastrointestinal fistulae are a challenging clinical problem caused by a broad spectrum of factors. The following images illustrate their findings. (A) Tracheoesophageal fistulae may be caused by infections such as tuberculosis and fungi, radiation, trauma, and tumors. (B) Postoperative gastropleural fistula (white arrow) after gastric sleeve surgery. (C) Enteroenteric fistula in Crohn disease. (D) Distal esophageal rupture in Boerhaave syndrome, partially closed by a fully covered self-expanding metal stent that now migrated to the stomach. In this case the SEMS was pulled back proximally and anchored with an over the scope clips. (E) Gastrocolonic fistula many years after gastrojejunostomy. (F) Gastrocutaneous fistula after removing percutaneous gastrostomy tube.

Classification of gastrointestinal fistulas and leaks

- **Organ/Location**
  - **Esophageal**
  - **Gastric**
  - **Small bowel**
  - **Colon**
  - **Pancreatobiliary**
- **Type**
  - **Entero-cutaneous**
  - **Entero-enteric**
  - **Entero-vesical**
  - **Esophago-tracheal**
  - **Entero-peritoneal**
- **Mechanism**
  - Traumatic (trauma/surgery)
  - Inflammatory (IBD, vasculitis)
  - Neoplastic
  - Radiation
- **Size**
  - Diminutive: 1–2 mm
  - Small: 2–6 mm
  - Medium: 6–12 mm
  - Large: >12 mm
- **Complexity**
  - Simple
  - Complex

Fig. 2. Classification of fistulae based on cause, location, duration, and size. This classification may help in deciding endoscopic versus surgical closure and the use of specific therapies and devices, including glues, clips, and stents.

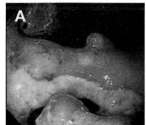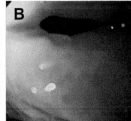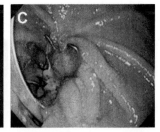

Fig. 3. It is important to recognize that some fistula or perforations may be impossible to close endoscopically due to its large size, presence of fibrosis, ongoing inflammation, complexity, or awkward location. (A) Large rectovaginal fistula. (B) Radiation-induced fibrotic tracheoesophageal fistula. (C) Small bowel fistula in a patient with Takayasu arteritis.

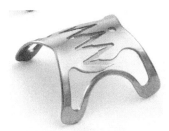

Fig. 4. The over the scope clips has various sizes and teeth configurations. The presence of sharp teeth improves anchoring. Despite its tight apposition capabilities, the space left in between the teeth allows for blood circulation, avoiding necrosis. (*Courtesy of* Ovesco Endoscopy AG, Tübingen, Germany; with permission.)

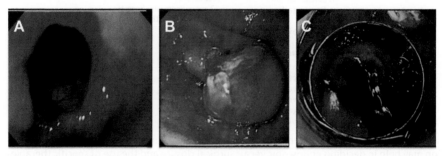

Fig. 5. Acute duodenal bulb perforation due to an endoscopic ultrasound scope (*A*). This type of perforation may be closed immediately with 11 or 12 mm over the scope clips (ie, 11/6t, 12/6t) (*B, C*). In this patient an immediate endoscopic retrograde cholangiopancreatography (ERCP) following endoscopic closure of the perforation was possible and essential to treat acute cholangitis.

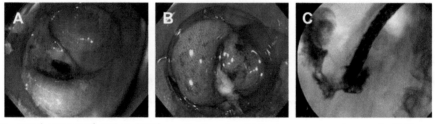

Fig. 6. Subacute perforation. (*A*) The patient underwent colonoscopy and presented 14 hours after discharge. Traditionally, patients with these types of perforation had to undergo immediate surgery. (*B*) In this case successful endoscopic closure was achieved with a 12/6t over the scope clips. (*C*) We always use water-soluble contrast delivered through the scope to verify closure of the gastrointestinal defect.

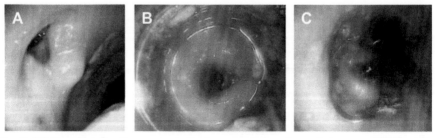

Fig. 7. (*A*) Rectal perforation as a result of mechanical endoscopic trauma. (*B*) When the diameter of the defect is less than 12 to 15 mm the primary closure may be applying suction technique (similar to using a banding device). (*C*) The tissue was nicely engulfed during suction and is now tightly trapped by the over the scope clips.

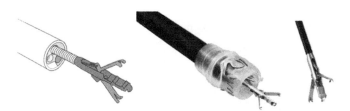

Fig. 8. When lesions are larger than 15 mm or seem complex or are located in difficult locations, the success of closure can be improved by using special grasping forceps (Twin Grasper, Ovesco, Tübingen). This twin grasping forceps is a unique invention, with 2 grasping arms acting individually. The 2 grasping arms act independently and are controlled separately with the handle of the forceps. The first step involves opening one arm, approaching one edge of the perforation or leak, and then closing the arm. The second arm is then opened and the forceps directed at the other edge of the perforation. Once the edge is grasped the arm is closed. Now both arms of the forceps are closed. The forceps is pulled back into the scope, tenting the grasped edges. Once both the distal tip of the forceps and the tented tissue are inside of the transparent cap holding the clip, the clip is fired (ie, released). The tissue at the base of the tented tissue is tightly grasped by the released over the scope clips, closing the perforation. (*Courtesy of* Ovesco Endoscopy AG, Tübingen, Germany; with permission.)

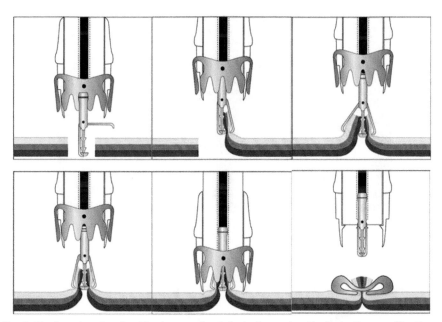

Fig. 9. The key steps involved in closure of a defect when using the Twin Grasper. The tissue is tightly grasped and gently pulled toward the scope and inside the distal cap, on which the clip is loaded. Once the tissue (and the forceps tip) is inside of the cap, the clip is released around the tissue. The tissue is then released from the grasper. (*Courtesy of* Ovesco Endoscopy AG, Tübingen, Germany; with permission.)

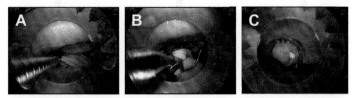

Fig. 10. In order to become proficient, we recommend to become familiar in advanced closing techniques by practicing in experimental models, such as in this ex-vivo pig stomach model, which they developed. (*A*) Twin Grasper used to catch the tissue. (*B*) The clip has been released and the perforation is successfully closed. (*C*) View of the clip on the perforation site.

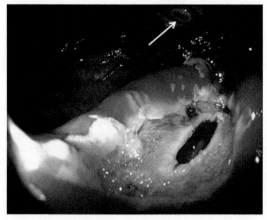

Fig. 11. After mucosectomy a perforation was noticed. The white arrow shows the reverse target sign.

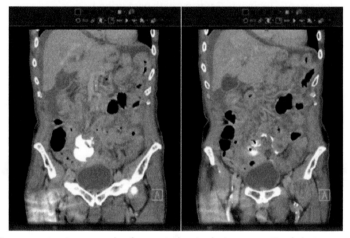

Fig. 12. On computer tomography free extraluminal air was noticed, but no ascites. The video shows the key steps described in Figs. 7–9.

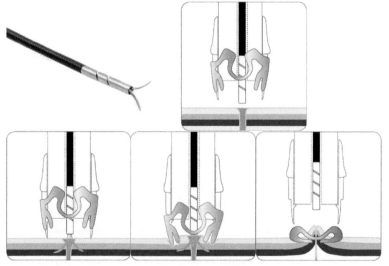

Fig. 13. Another device used to close complex fistulae and dehiscences is the anchoring forceps. (*Courtesy of* Ovesco Endoscopy AG, Tübingen, Germany; with permission.)

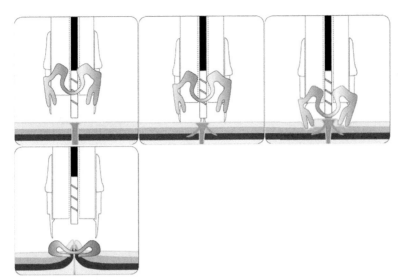

Fig. 14. The concept of closure is similar as to when using the Twin Grasper: the device helps pull the grasped tissue into the cap, and then the clip is released toward the base of the tented tissue, thus closing the defect. (*Courtesy of* Ovesco Endoscopy AG, Tübingen, Germany; with permission.)

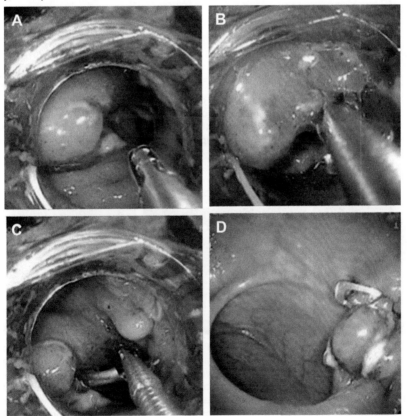

Fig. 15. Endoscopic closure of a complex colon perforation using the Twin Grasper (*A*). We do not recommend closing most colon perforation using the suctioning technique alone, as occasionally adjacent organs such as the ureter or small bowel may be unintentionally suctioned into the clip. By using the grasping forceps one ensures holding only the edges of the intended tissue to be trapped within the over the scope clips (*B, C, D*). (*Courtesy of* Ovesco Endoscopy AG, Tübingen, Germany.)

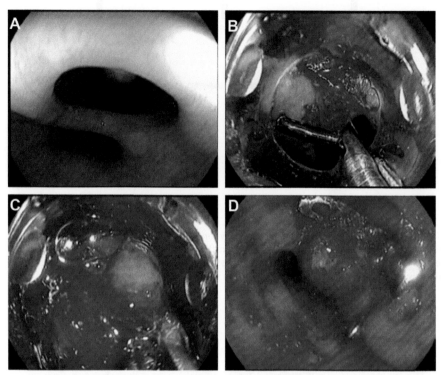

Fig. 16. Complex esophagotracheal fistula (*A*) closed using Twin Grasper (*B*) and a 12/6t over the scope clips (*C, D*). Especially in these types of esophagotracheal fistulae, suctioning tissue into the cap is impossible, as suction removes the air from the bronchial tree. Suctioning maneuver may thus be counterproductive, dropping the patient's tidal volume to dangerous levels.

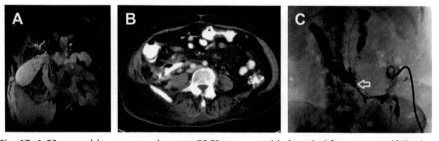

Fig. 17. A 60-year-old woman underwent ERCP at an outside hospital for suspected bile duct stones. (*A*) A common bile duct (CBD) stricture was noted and a 7Fr × 15 cm long plastic stent was inserted. She subsequently underwent laparoscopic cholecystectomy for cholelithiasis. Postoperatively she developed an intraabdominal abscess, believed to have resulted from surgery. (*B*) However, a duodenal perforation induced by the biliary stent was noticed. (*C*) The abscess was drained percutaneously inserting one drainage catheter into the collection but the fistulous leak and perforation persisted (yellow arrow). In the meantime a diagnosis of cholangiocarcinoma was confirmed and surgical resection was planned. However, the presence of a perforation and the persistent abscess would have implied a more aggressive and riskier surgical approach.

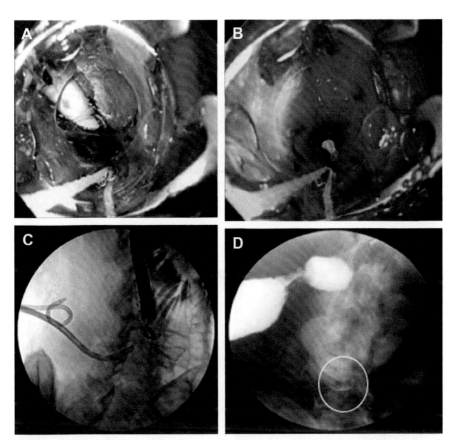

Fig. 18. Part 2 of the case presented in Fig. 17. (*A*) An endoscopic closure of the perforation using an 11/6t over the scope clips was performed. The fistulous perforation was approached under direct endoscopic visualization. (*B*) The 11/6t over the scope clips was placed against the perforation, the tissue was suctioned inside of the cap, and the clip was released. The endoscopic procedure lasted 8 minutes. (*C*) Intraendoscopic soluble contrast study confirmed adequate closure of the perforation. (*D*) The clip is nicely attached to the duodenal wall (yellow circle).

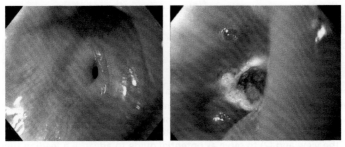

Fig. 19. Long-standing esophagotracheal fistula may be more difficult to close endoscopically. By applying thermal energy (eg, argon plasma coagulation) to the borders of the fistulous orifice the chances of permanent tissue apposition may increase. It is more likely that acutely damaged tissue will release fibrinogen, thrombin, and other factors necessary to start a clot and activate procollagen IV and fibrosis.

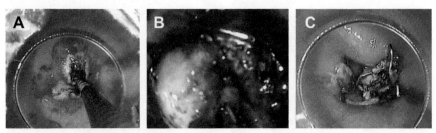

Fig. 20. Thermocoagulation of the fistulous orifice may also be accomplished with hot biopsy forceps (*A, B, C*). (*Courtesy of* Ovesco Endoscopy AG, Tübingen, Germany.)

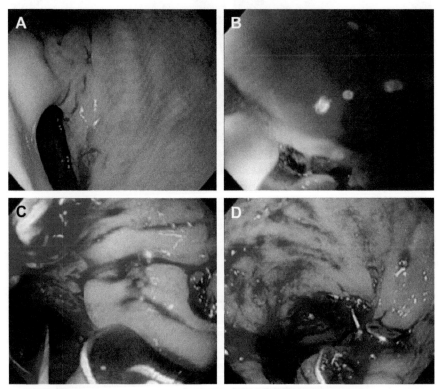

Fig. 21. This case showing the closure of a complex esophagotracheal fistula (*A*) shows 2 technical tricks. (*B*) Application of argon plasma coagulation. (*C*) In order to keep the luminal view a wire was advanced into the stomach. The wire serves to main purposes: (1) to keep the view and (2) to serve as potential guide to advance a feeding tube or nasogastric catheter in case of a stenosis after clip closure. (*D*) In this case there was immediate no postclosure stenosis. Thus, the wire was removed.

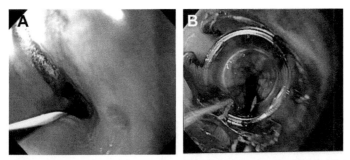

Fig. 22. Large laceration of the trachea, exposing the endotracheal balloon. (*A*) A wire was placed to advance a self-expanding metal stent. (*B*) The wire was also useful to keep the luminal view.

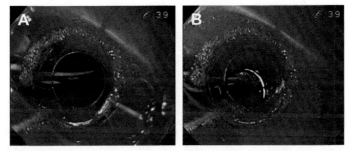

Fig. 23. (*A*) Wire and nasogastric tube. (*B*) over the scope clips closure of a fistula. The lumen was stenosed after clip application. However, the nasogastric tube bridged the stenosis and served as feeding tube during the next 48 hours.

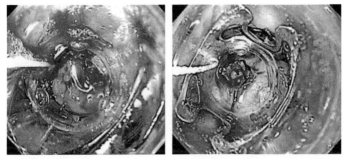

Fig. 24. Occasionally, fibrotic fistulae may be very friable and bleed, thus obscuring the file of view. Sometimes, the small fistulous opening may disappear to the examining eye.

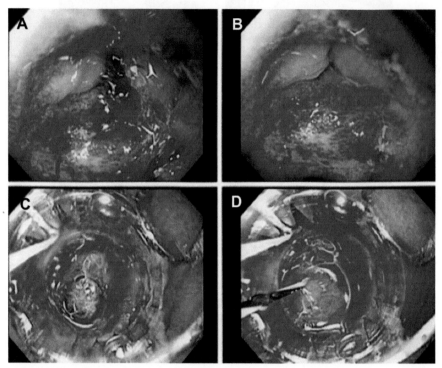

Fig. 25. Small fistulous opening surrounded by massive edema (*A*), fibrosis (*B*), and friable tissue (*C*). Inserting a wire (*D*) into the fistulous tract may aid in keeping the defect in view. This maneuver allows for proper en face approach with the cap and clip, thus improving the chances of targeted closure.

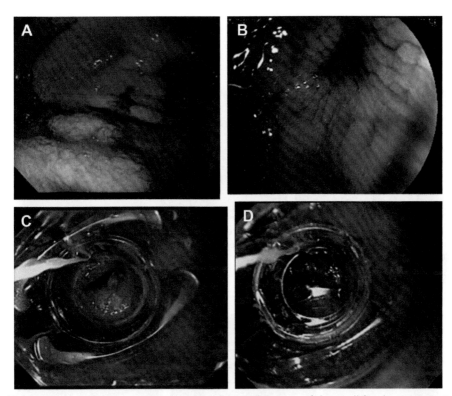

Fig. 26. The use of chromoendoscopy may improve detection of the small fistulae. A patient who had suffered from gunshot wound to the abdomen was fed through a gastrostomy tube for several months. Once his ability to tolerate oral intake improved, the tube was pulled. However, a gastrocutaneous fistula persisted for 5 months. On esophagogastroduodenoscopy it was impossible to locate the fistula. (*A*) A biliary catheter was inserted percutaneously through the skin and indigo carmine was injected. (*B*) The dye appeared in a conglomerate of folds, exposing the stomach side of the gastrocutaneous fistula. (*C*) The over the scope clips clip apparatus could be targeted on top of the fistulous opening. (*D*) The fistula was successfully closed with a 12/6gc over the scope clips.

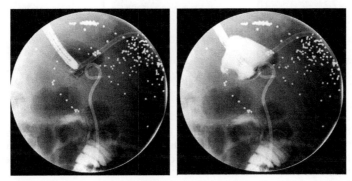

Fig. 27. The through the scope water-soluble contrast application demonstrated complete closure of the fistula. Note the large amount of gunshot pellets remaining in the patient's abdomen.

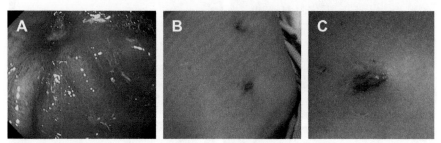

Fig. 28. Persistent gastrocutaneous fistulae are not uncommon (*A, B*). Usually, these fistulae are fibrotic and occur in patients who suffered recurrent infections of the gastrostomy site (*C*).

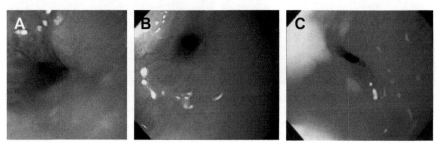

Fig. 29. Spectrum of persistent gastrocutaneous fistulae (*A, B, C*). The fistula is often very small, but recalcitrant.

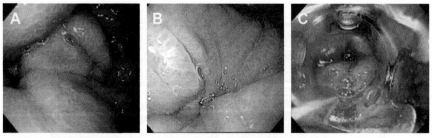

Fig. 30. A trick to find these persistent fistulae is to search for thick and convergent gastric folds (*A*). The fistula is located at the base of these enlarged folds (*B*). By using the folds as linear guide, it is possible to push the cap and clip onto the orifice (*C*) and then release the over the scope clips onto the hole.

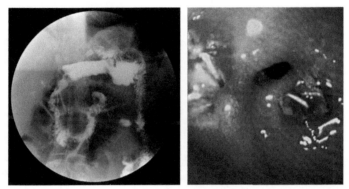

Fig. 31. Gastrogastric fistula may result in bloating, diarrhea, and weight gain in patients with Roux-en-Y gastric bypass. The diagnosis of these fistulae is done by upper gastrointestinal series and endoscopy.

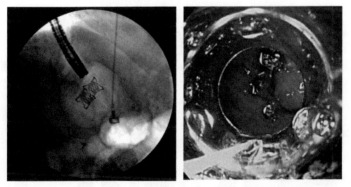

Fig. 32. Double clipping approach. Two 11/6t over the scope clips were necessary to close this fistula.

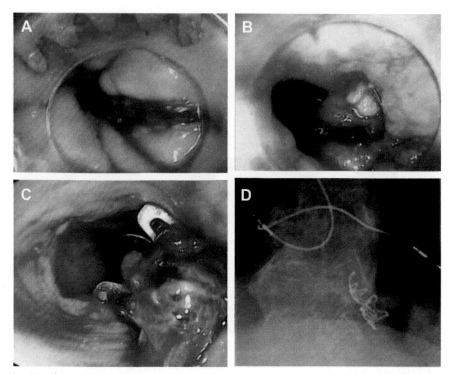

Fig. 33. This patient with iatrogenic esophageal perforation (*A*) necessitated 2 over the scope clips to close the large defect in upper esophagus (*B, C, D*).

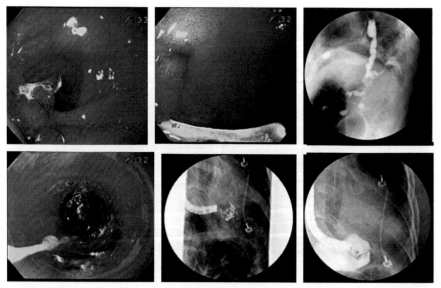

Fig. 34. A 50-year-old woman with gastric sleeve surgery, gastroperitoneo-pleural fistula, abdominal sepsis developed a gastroperitoneopleural fistula. The fistula was initially partially closed using a stent. The fully covered self-expanding metal stent was removed and 2 over the scope clips were applied. Successful closure was achieved. This was confirmed by injection of water-soluble contrast.

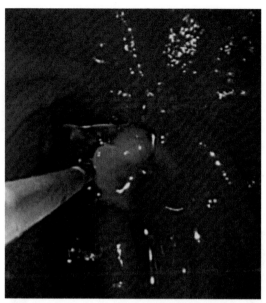

Fig. 35. Combination of over the scope clips and injection of fibrin glue to close an enterocutaneous fistula in a patient with small bowel Crohn disease.

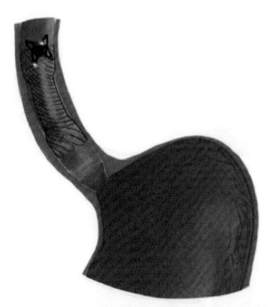

Fig. 36. A typical use of over the scope clips "beyond its standard use" is anchoring of fully covered self-expanding metal stents. Large esophageal defects, including Boerhaave syndrome, esophageal perforations, and postoperative dehiscence of anastomosis or esophagotracheal lacerations often mandate the initial placement of a fully covered self-expandable metal stent to bridge the defect, keep the lumen patent, and occlude the defect. The stent may result in complete healing and closure of the defect or at least decrease in size to allow subsequent closure with clips, including over the scope clips (Drawing by: Kirsten O. Tucker).

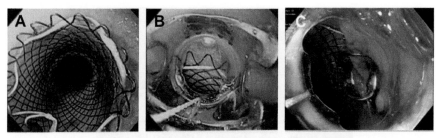

Fig. 37. The over the scope clips has more occlusive power than standard through the scope clips. The cohesive force of a closed clip approaches 6 N. The photos show appropriate anchoring of a fully covered self-expanding metal stent (fcSEMS) (*A, B, C*).

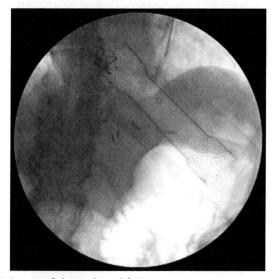

Fig. 38. Radiologic image of the anchored fcSEMS.

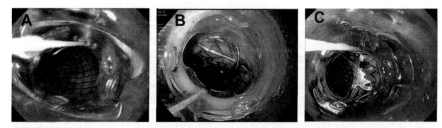

Fig. 39. When anchoring fcSEMS, it is important to catch only the most proximal part of the stent (*A*) and avoid pushing the stent distally while maneuvering the scope (*B, C*).

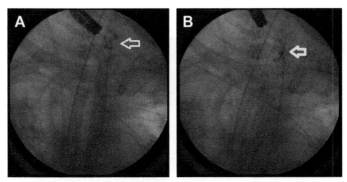

Fig. 40. Pulling the big wheel back on the handle of the scope will move the tip of the scope toward a perpendicular position within the lumen, allowing for better positioning of the cap and clip. The yellow arrows show the clip. (*A*) Before release. (*B*) After being fired.

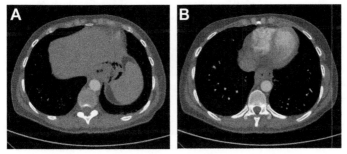

Fig. 41. (*A*) A 45-year-old alcoholic patient with massive nausea and retching developed a Boerhaave syndrome. (*B*) Notice the double barrel sign.

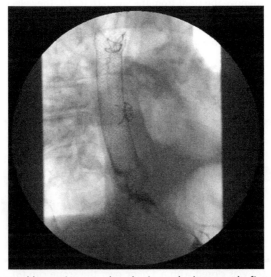

Fig. 42. The esophageal laceration was closed using a dual approach: first an over the scope clips was applied, with partial closure and then a fcSEMS was placed to close the wound and bridge the lesion and maintain the lumen. The fcSEMS was anchored with an 11/6t over the scope clips.

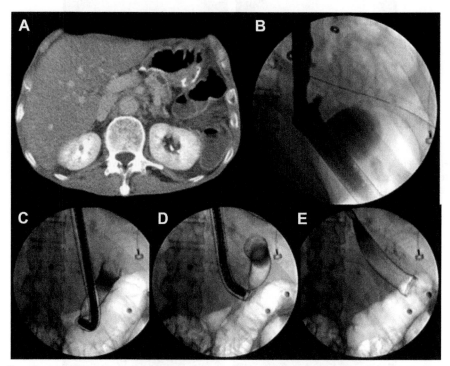

Fig. 43. A 50-year-old man with Boerhaave syndrome underwent placement of fcSEMS to treat his condition (A). The fcSEMS resulted in partial closure of the perforation, but it migrated into the stomach (B). A fistulous tract (esophagopleural fistula) was evident. We used an overtube to remove the stent from the stomach (C, D). They elected to use an overtube to prevent damage from stent scratching the damaged and frail gastroesophageal junction (GEJ), where the fistula was present. The overtube served as a giant "working channel" to remove the foreign body and at the same time protect the esophagus and GEJ (E).

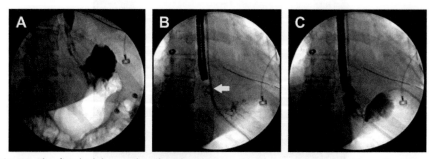

Fig. 44. The fistula (A) was closed with a 12/6gc over the scope clip (B). The yellow arrow shows the over the scope clip. Water-soluble contrast examination confirmed complete closure (C).

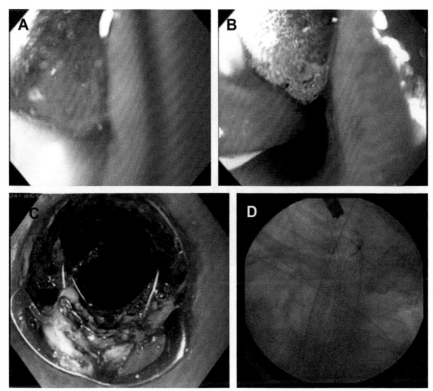

Fig. 45. Large tracheal injury (*A*). The endotracheal tube balloon clearly protrudes into the esophagus (*B*). This large fistula could not be closed with clips. Therefore, a lifesaving fcSEMS was used to bridge the defect. The fcSEMS anchored with an 11/3t over the scope clips (*C, D*).

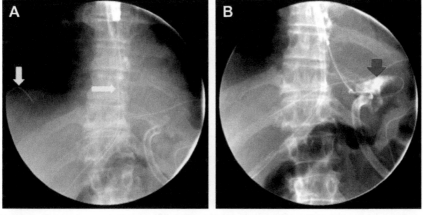

Fig. 46. Endoscopic reanastomosis of a disrupted gastroesophageal junction (Figs. 46–50). A 61-year-old patient with esophageal cancer suffered from an esophageal perforation after placement of a fully covered SEMS. The stent was removed and the patient underwent laparotomy and thoracotomy. A gastrostomy tube was placed surgically. On repeat imaging, the esophagus and stomach were nearly completely disrupted and the patient was deemed not a good surgical candidate. (*A*) During endoscopy no lumen could be found distally. A wire traveled preferentially into the chest cavity (*yellow arrows*). (*B*) Water-soluble contrast injection demonstrated trickling of contrast into the stomach (red arrow).

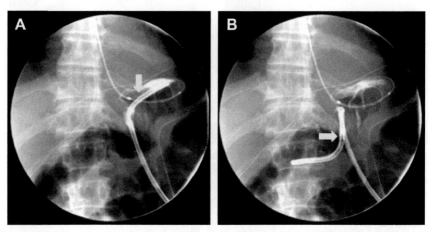

Fig. 47. The gastrostomy was removed and an ultraslim gastroscope (*A*) was inserted into the stomach to visualize the trickling of Indigo carmine injected through the upper gastroscope. Once a potential communication was confirmed, a 0.035-in guidewire was then advanced into the stomach under constant ultraslim gastroscope visualization (*B*). The yellow arrows show the tip of the ultraslim gastroscope, which had been inserted through the gastrostomy opening.

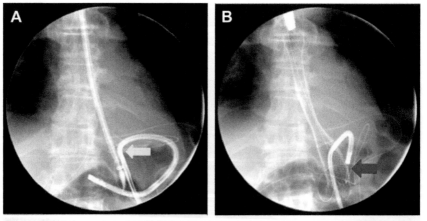

Fig. 48. A fully covered SEMS (*A*) was placed through esophagogastroduodenoscopy into the stomach and deployed after visual confirmation (*B*) of intraluminal placement with the ultraslim gastroscope (*red arrow*). The yellow arrow shows the distal part of the stent before deployment.

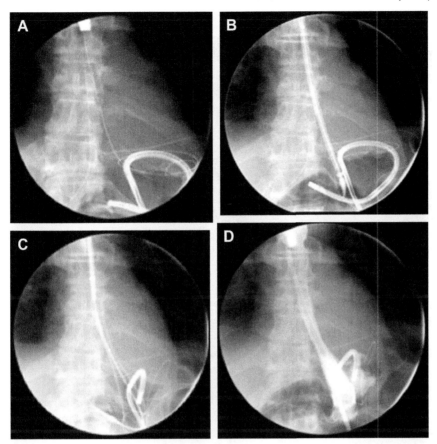

Fig. 49. A second fully covered SEMS was placed into the previous SEMS to allow for complete bridging of the perforation and tumor (*A, B, C*). An over the scope clips was attached to the proximal end of the second stent in order to anchor it and prevent migration. Injection of water-soluble contrast confirmed position of both stents without extraluminal contrast leak (*D*).

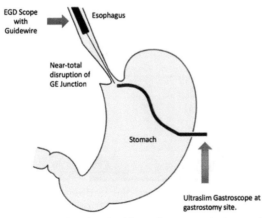

Fig. 50. Endoscopic reanastomosis using double-endoscope technique, wires, stent, and over the scope clips.

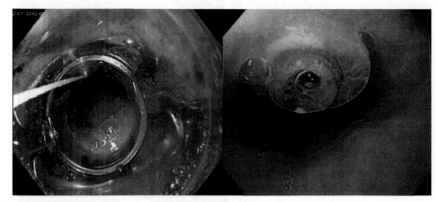

Fig. 51. Insertion of the loaded over the scope clips into the esophagus is quite easy. However, careful attention must be paid to stenosis, rings, diverticula, and foreign bodies such as voice devices.

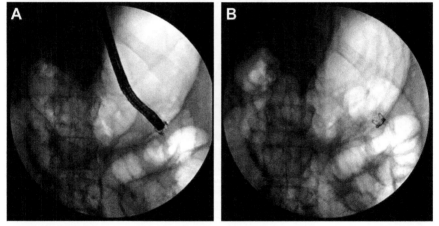

Fig. 52. (*A*) Radiologic visualization of endoscope with over the scope clips. (*B*) Deployed over the scope clips.

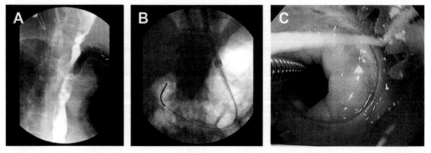

Fig. 53. (*A*) Placement of an over the scope clips to close a gastrocutaneous fistula was potentially impeded by an esophageal stricture. (*B*) Gently dilate the stenosis. (*C*) The wire was left in place and served as a stabilizing and visual guide while advancing the scope loaded with over the scope clips through the esophagus into the stomach, to successfully treat the gastrocutaneous fistula.

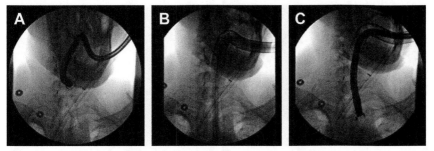

Fig. 54. The loaded scope with over the scope clips could not be advanced into the stomach due to an upper esophageal stenosis (*A*). The stenosis was bridged by using an overtube (*B*). The scope loaded with an 11/6t over the scope clips could now be advanced into the overtube through the esophagus into the stomach, to successfully treat the gastrocutaneous fistula (*C*). On another occasion we had a patient with bleeding peptic ulcer and an esophageal stenosis. The overtube technique allowed for the passage of the loaded scope with over the scope clips to treat the ulcer.

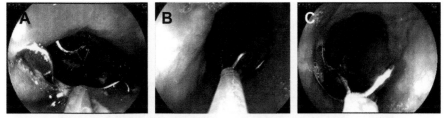

Fig. 55. Endoscopic removal of over the scope clips. The base of the clip is injected with saline and epinephrine solution, creating a submucosal cushion (*A*). Then the cushion is circumferentially incised. Then a snare is placed around the raised clip and removed it with cold or hot technique (*B, C*).

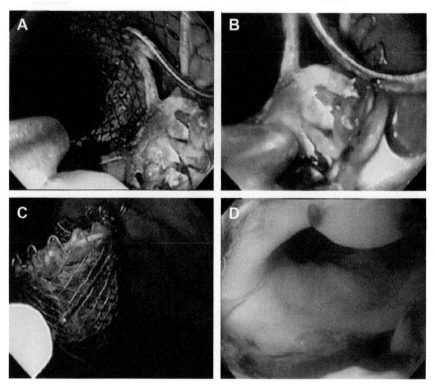

Fig. 56. Endoscopic removal of over the scope clips. The base of the clip is injected with saline and epinephrine solution, creating a submucosal cushion (*A*). Then the cushion is circumferentially incised. Then a snare is placed around the raised clip and removed it with cold or hot technique (*B, C*). Inspection of the previous clip site (*D*).

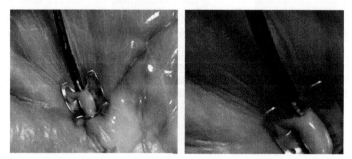

Fig. 57. Removal of an over the scope clips using the remove DC Cutter, which uses electrofragmentation. (*Courtesy of* Ovesco Endoscopy AG, Tübingen, Germany.)

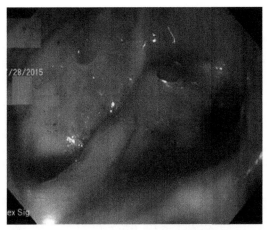

Fig. 58. Combination therapy for over the scope clips and Endo-SPONGE to heal large colorectal anastomotic leaks (Figs. 58–61). Large dehiscence after colorectal surgery for diverticulitis.

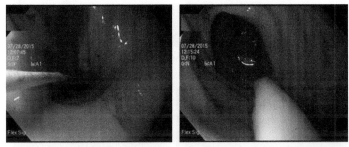

Fig. 59. A rectal tube was placed to guarantee stool passage and decompress the colon.

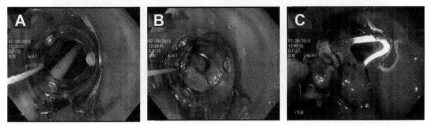

Fig. 60. Partial closure of the anastomotic leak using two 12/6t over the scope clips (*A, B, C*).

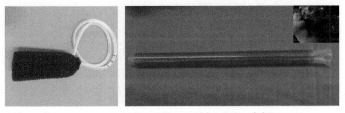

Fig. 61. Insertion of a sponge system to suction and heal the dehiscence.

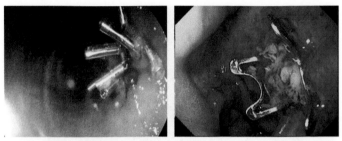

Fig. 62. Although the over the scope clips is currently used as first-line therapy for peptic ulcer bleeding, it is also quite useful for complex peptic ulcer lesions. Not only is it faster to
apply, but over the scope clips application is easier than placing multiple clips.

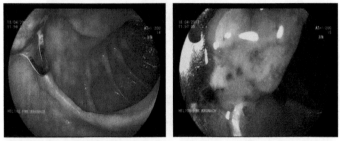

Fig. 63. Ulcers not reachable by traditional through the scope clip may be treated better
with over the scope clips device.

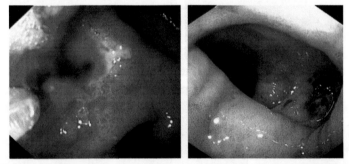

Fig. 64. Whereas traditional endoscopic therapy for bleeding peptic ulcer is accomplished
with dual therapy, application of over the scope clips may suffice as single therapy.

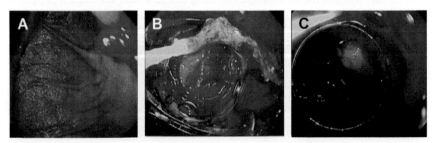

Fig. 65. The contraction ability of over the scope clips is ideal to compress large bleeding vessels. (A) Bleeding dieulafoy. (B) Approach with the clip. (C) Hemostasis.

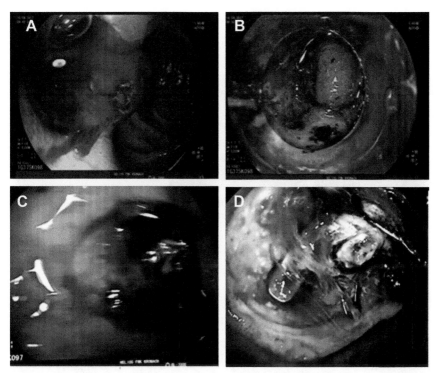

Fig. 66. During endoscopy of bleeding peptic ulcer, when the visual field is obscured (*A*), us-ing an over the scope clip may prove advantageous. The water flushing through the scope channel will come out the loaded transparent cap attached at the tip of the scope (*B*). This will allow for targeted cleaning of the ulcer base, expose the vessel (*C*), and fire the clip onto it (*D*).

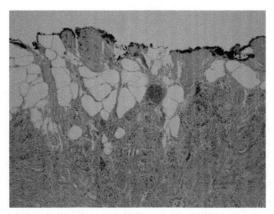

Fig. 67. One of the latest "beyond standard uses" of the over the scope clips is for full-thickness resection of endoluminal gastrointestinal tumors such as this neuroendocrine tumor.

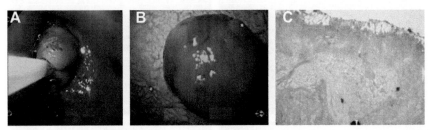

Fig. 68. Endoscopic full-thickness resection of a leiomyoma of the esophagus (*A*) using traditional suck and release technique, with snaring of the tumor above the clip (*B*, *C*).

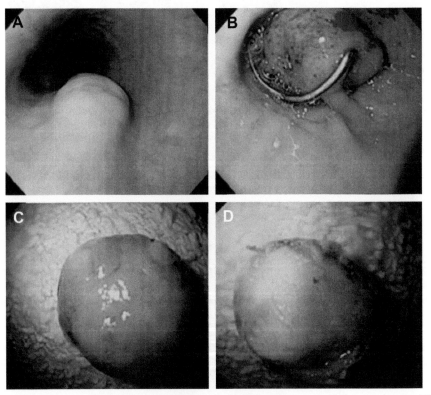

Fig. 69. Endoscopic full-thickness resection of an Abrikosoff tumor of the esophagus. (*A*) Abrikosoff's tumor. (*B*) Clip applied. (*C*) Resected tumor. (*D*) Ventral side of the tumor.

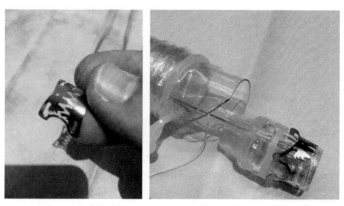

Fig. 70. The new endoscopic full-thickness resection device is one of the safest and most efficient methods to resect tumors up to 20 mm in size. (Photos by Klaus Mönkemüller; over the scope clips device *Courtesy of* Ovesco Endoscopy AG, Tübingen, Germany.)

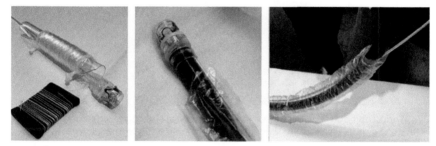

Fig. 71. The cap with loaded clip is attached to the tip of the scope. The snare runs along the distal cap, outside of the scope, along an accessory catheter (extra working channel). Therefore, a sheet is placed over the scope and catheter, to allow for easier insertion and maneuverability within the colon. (*Courtesy of* Ovesco Endoscopy AG, Tübingen, Germany.)

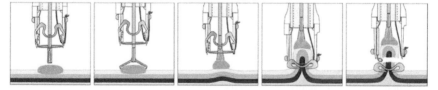

Fig. 72. Scheme showing the steps involved in endoscopic full thickness resection. The lesion is slowly and gently pulled with the forceps into the distal cap. Then the lesion is tightly grasped with a snare. The clip is released. Then electrosurgical current is applied to the snare and the lesion is resected. (*Courtesy of* Ovesco Endoscopy AG, Tübingen, Germany.)

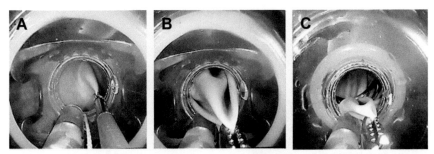

Fig. 73. Endoscopic view of steps involved in full-thickness resection (*A, B, C*). Notice the white ring located on the cap. If the ring is moved distally, then the clip has been released (*C*). Once this is visualized the snare grasping the lesion can be energized with electrocautery to effect a resection. (*A*) Catching lesion. (*B*) Gently pulling lesion. (*C*) Snaring of lesion.

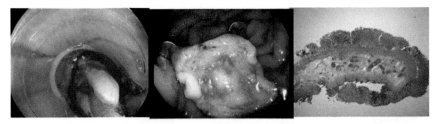

Fig. 74. Endoscopic full-thickness resection is not only useful to resect tumors but also to investigate the entire wall of the gastrointestinal tract such as in this patient with Hirschsprung disease.

Table 1 Endoscopic treatment of nonvariceal gastrointestinal bleeding	
Traditional approach	
Injection	Epinephrine, polidocanol, fibrin glue, histoacryl
Thermal therapies	Argon plasma coagulation, heater probes, monopolar, bipolar (gold, silver, BICAP)
Mechanical	Through the scope (TTS)—hemoclips, endoscopic band ligation
Emerging Treatments	
Injection	EUS-guided angiotherapy
Thermal therapies	Coagulation grasper, radiofrequency ablation, cryotherapy
Mechanical	Over the scope clips (Ovesco over-the-scope-clips, Padlock), suturing system (Apollo) anchor system (prototypes), flexible linear stapler (experimental)
Topical	Hemospray, Endoclot, Pure-Stat, Ankaferd Blood Stopper, oxidized cellulose

ACKNOWLEDGMENTS

We thank Kirsten O. Tucker (Phoenix, Arizona, United States of America) and Borja Martínez-Alcalá (Seville, Spain) for their expertise and professional input and design of the graphics and artistic figures. We thank Ovesco Endoscopy AG, Tübingen, Germany for providing additional material and graphics. As per policy of Gastrointestinal Endoscopy Clinics of North America we have placed a manufacturer courtesy line at the end of graphics/figure legends mentioning or showing that manufacturer's product.

DISCLOSURE

K. Mönkemüller has been speaker/consultant for Cook Medical, USA and Ovesco, Germany; A.R. Schmidt has been speaker/consultant for Ovesco, Germany; T. Kratt has been speaker/consultant for Ovesco, Germany; A. Martínez-Alcalá does not have any conflicts of interest to declare.

SUPPLEMENTARY DATA

Supplementary video related to this article can be found at https://doi.org/10.1016/j.giec.2019.09.003.

REFERENCES

1. Mönkemüller K, Peter S, Toshniwal J, et al. Multipurpose use of the 'bear claw' (over-the-scope-clip system) to treat endoluminal gastrointestinal disorders. Dig Endosc 2014;26(3):350–7.
2. Mönkemüller K, Toshniwal J, Zabielski M. Utility of the "bear claw", or over-the-scope clip (over-the-scope-clips) system, to provide endoscopic hemostasis for bleeding posterior duodenal ulcers. Endoscopy 2012;44(Suppl 2 UCTN): E412–3.
3. Vormbrock K, Zabielski M, Mönkemüller K. Use of the "bear claw" (over-the-scope-clip) to achieve hemostasis of a large gastric ulcer with bleeding visible vessel. Gastrointest Endosc 2012;76(4):917–8.
4. von Renteln D, Denzer UW, Schachschal G, et al. Endoscopic closure of GI fistulae by using an over-the-scope clip (with videos). Gastrointest Endosc 2010;72:1289–96.
5. Sulz MC, Bertolini R, Frei R, et al. Multipurpose use of the over-the-scope-clip system ("Bear claw") in the gastrointestinal tract: Swiss experience in a tertiary center. World J Gastroenterol 2014;20(43):16287–92.
6. Honegger C, Valli PV, Wiegand N, et al. Establishment of Over-The-Scope-Clips (over-the-scope-clips®) in daily endoscopic routine. United European Gastroenterol J 2017;5(2):247–54.
7. Richter-Schrag HJ, Glatz T, Walker C, et al. First-line endoscopic treatment with over-the-scope clips significantly improves the primary failure and rebleeding rates in high-risk gastrointestinal bleeding: a single-center experience with 100 cases. World J Gastroenterol 2016;22(41):9162–71.
8. Wedi E, Fischer A, Hochberger J, et al. Multicenter evaluation of first-line endoscopic treatment with the over-the-scope-clips in acute non-variceal upper gastrointestinal bleeding and comparison with the Rockall cohort: the FLETRock study. Surg Endosc 2017. https://doi.org/10.1007/s00464-017-5678-7.

9. Skinner M, Gutierrez JP, Neumann H, et al. Over-the-scope clip placement is effective rescue therapy for severe acute upper gastrointestinal bleeding. Endosc Int Open 2014;2:E37–40.

10. Chan SM, Chiu PW, Teoh AY, et al. Use of the Over-The-Scope Clip for treatment of refractory upper gastrointestinal bleeding: a case series. Endoscopy 2014; 46(5):428–31.

11. Manta R, Galloro G, Mangiavillano B, et al. Over-the-scope clip (over-the-scope-clips) represents an effective endoscopic treatment for acute GI bleeding after failure of conventional techniques. Surg Endosc 2013;27(9):3162–4.

12. Mudumbi S, Velazquez-Aviña J, Neumann H, et al. Anchoring of self-expanding metal stents using the over-the-scope clip, and a technique for subsequent removal. Endoscopy 2014;46:1106–9.

13. Mudumbi S, Mönkemüller K. Endoscopic re-anastomosis of esophagus and stomach using dual endoscope technique with two fully covered metal stents and over-the-scope-clip. Dig Endosc 2014;26(3):493–4.

14. Sarker S, Gutierrez JP, Council L, et al. Over-the-scope clip-assisted method for resection of full-thickness submucosal lesions of the gastrointestinal tract. Endoscopy 2014;46(9):758–61.

15. Gutierrez JP, Sarker S, Wilcox M, et al. "Clip and let go" for resection of duodenal carcinoid: a new technique using the over-the-scope-clip. Endoscopy 2014; 46(Suppl 1 UCTN):E61.

16. Mönkemüller K, Sarker S, Baig KR. Endoscopic creation of an omental patch with an over-the-scope clip system after endoscopic excavation and resection of a large gastrointestinal stromal tumor of the stomach. Endoscopy 2014;46(Suppl 1 UCTN):E451–2.

17. Abe S, Council L, Cui X, et al. Endoscopic resection and enucleation of gastric submucosal tumor facilitated by subsequent closure of incision using over-the-scope clip. Endoscopy 2015;47(Suppl 1 UCTN):E153–4.

18. Manno M, Mangiafico S, Caruso A, et al. First-line endoscopic treatment with over-the-scope-clips in patients with high-risk non-variceal upper gastrointestinal bleeding: preliminary experience in 40 cases. Surg Endosc 2016;30(5):2026–9.

19. Wedi E, von Renteln D, Gonzalez S, et al. Use of the over-the-scope-clip (over-the-scope-clips) in non-variceal upper gastrointestinal bleeding in patients with severe cardiovascular comorbidities: a retrospective study. Endosc Int Open 2017;5(9):E875–82.

20. Lamberts R, Koch A, Binner C, et al. Use of over-the-scope clips (over-the-scope-clips) for hemostasis in gastrointestinal bleeding in patients under antithrombotic therapy. Endosc Int Open 2017;5(5):E324–30.

Complications with Over the Scope Clip

How Can We Prevent It?

Ravishankar Asokkumar, MBBS, MD, MRCP[a,b,*],
Yung-Ka Chin, MD, MBChB, MRCP[a], Roy Soetikno, MD, MS[c,d]

KEYWORDS

- Over the scope clip • Misplacement • Treatment failure • Complication • Safety tips

KEY POINTS

- Over the scope clip is safe and effective for the treatment of gastrointestinal bleeding, perforation, and fistulas.
- The occurrence of complication with over the scope clip application is rare and could be avoided.
- Precision during clip placement and appropriate use of accessories would prevent serious adverse events.

INTRODUCTION

In the past, flexible endoscopic methods to treat refractory nonvariceal gastrointestinal (GI) bleeding, perforation, GI leaks, and fistula were limited.[1] In many such cases, invasive and morbid surgeries were performed to achieve symptom control and cure. With the introduction of the over the scope clip (OTSC; Ovesco Endoscopy AG, Tuebingen, Germany), treatment of such lesions from within the bowel lumen has become a possibility, and the need for surgical intervention has declined.[2] The ease of use, its resemblance to the band ligation device, and the shorter learning curve has made the OTSC system popular and readily adopted in clinical practice. The device is currently approved for the treatment of bleeding (vessel <2 mm), closure of perforation, mucosal defects (<3 cm), and endoscopic marking.[3] There is accumulating evidence expanding the utility of OTS clip beyond the approved indications.[4]

Multiple studies, from both tertiary academic centers and community practice, have established its safety, efficacy, and durability as compared with conventional

Disclosure Statement: The authors have no disclosures.
[a] Department of Gastroenterology and Hepatology, Singapore General Hospital, 20, College Road, Singapore 169586; [b] Bariatric Endoscopy Unit, HM Sanchinarro University Hospital, Madrid, Spain; [c] Advanced GI Endoscopy, 2490 Hospital Drive, Suite 211, El Camino Hospital, Mountain View, CA 94040, USA; [d] The University of Indonesia, Jakarta, Indonesia
* Corresponding author. Singapore General Hospital, 20, College Road, Singapore 169586.
E-mail address: ravishnkr03@gmail.com

Gastrointest Endosc Clin N Am 30 (2020) 75–89
https://doi.org/10.1016/j.giec.2019.08.003
1052-5157/20/© 2019 Elsevier Inc. All rights reserved.

therapy.[5–9] The OTSC, unlike the traditional hemostatic clips, can capture a large amount of tissue and stay secure, providing a lasting effect. However, this property of OTSC can also make removal of the clip arduous when misplaced. Since its widespread adoptions and use, reports on complications after OTSC are emerging. The reported complication rate with OTSC is approximately 1.7%, and the risk of severe adverse event was 0.6% (**Fig. 1**).[9] Most of these complications can be managed conservatively, whereas the serious adverse events require surgery. In this article, we will discuss complications that may occur with the OTSC system, provide measures to mitigate such complications, and describe techniques to remove the OTSC.

KNOWING THE DEVICE

The OTSC applicator system consists of a distal transparent applicator cap mounted with the clip, a threaded wire, and a hand-wheel release mechanism. The technique of installation and application is similar to the band ligation device used for treating esophageal varices. The OTSC is made up of nitinol, a biocompatible, MRI conditional, superelastic, and shape-memory alloy. The clip is premounted on the applicator cap with its jaws open at 90°, as opposed to its neutral closed state. It provides the compression energy at the jaws when released. Animal studies have shown that the closing force of the OTSC is around 8 to 9 N.[10]

The OTSC comes in 3 different sizes (11 mm, 12 mm, and 14 mm) and 3 tip designs suited for different indications. The atraumatic blunt type is used for tissue compression; the traumatic t-type with small spikes at the distal end is used for compression and anchoring, and the gc-type with long spikes is used for gastric wall closure. The depth of the cap can also be adjusted depending on the location of use to 3 or 6 mm (**Fig. 2**). The OTSC system also has 2 accessories to assist with clip deployment: (a) the OTSC twin grasper for approximating the gaping edges and (b) the OTSC anchor with a triprong design used for indurated and fibrotic tissue, which has 2 designs with different triprong widths (9 mm, 12 mm) and depths (2.5 mm, 4 mm) for use in the stomach and colon.

We strongly recommend being familiar with the device description and specifications to achieve success with OTSC use and avoid complications.

PREPROCEDURE PLANNING, CLIP SELECTION, AND TECHNIQUE

Choosing the appropriate OTSC size, type, and accessory in certain situations is critical for achieving technical success and avoiding misplacement. We recommend

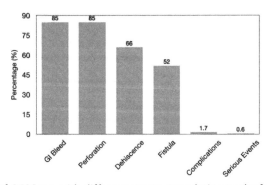

Fig. 1. Outcome of OTSC use with different causes. Cumulative results from 30 articles and 1517 patients showed the risk of complications and serious adverse events with over the scope clip is very low.

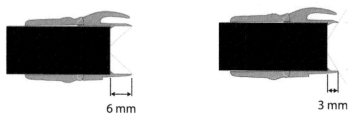

6 mm   3 mm

Fig. 2. The OTSC cap can be adjusted to 6 or 3 mm depending on the cause. The selection of the cap should be based on the lesion being treated.

using a therapeutic channel upper endoscope (3.7 mm) when using OTSC. It allows concurrent smooth use of the OTSC accessories and has adequate suction capability. We suggest using water-jet and carbon dioxide (CO_2) insufflation to visualize the target tissue before clip placement.[11]

We choose the clip size depending on the size of the target lesion/tissue (**Fig. 3**). A small clip for a large fibrotic and deep ulcer may be inadequate. We recommend using the medium-sized OTSC (12 mm), which in most instances, is adequate to treat the frequently encountered GI conditions. We use the traumatic type OTSC in chronic and fibrotic tissue and the atraumatic type for other tissue. Similarly, we also adjust the depth of the cap depending on the location of its use. We adjust the depth of the cap to 3 mm for most targeted tissue because it prevents capture of excessive tissue. In situations, such as perforation, where more tissue grasping is required, we use the 6-mm deep cap.[11]

We deploy the OTSC using the suction technique or by using traction with the aid of an accessory. We position the target tissue within the perimeter of the cap and apply continuous suction to draw the tissue inside the cap and then deploy the clip for secure placement. In deep fibrotic tissue, where suction alone is not adequate, we use OTSC anchor to apply traction. The OTSC anchor when opened can pierce the muscularis propria and hook the tissue to allow firm traction inside the cap for clipping. Standardization of clip deployment techniques and training the assistants with OTSC accessories are essential for achieving consistent success with OTSC.

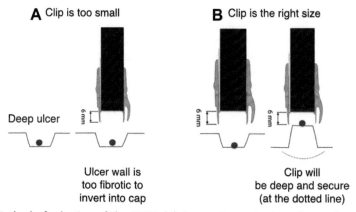

A Clip is too small   **B** Clip is the right size

Deep ulcer

Ulcer wall is
too fibrotic to
invert into cap

Clip will
be deep and secure
(at the dotted line)

Fig. 3. Method of selection of the OTSC. (*A*) Appropriate selection of over the scope clip based on ulcer dimension is important. A small-sized OTSC is ineffective in inverting a large ulcer and the vessel into the cap. (*B*) A large OTSC, matching the size of the ulcer, successfully inverted the ulcer with suction and clipped securely.

COMPLICATIONS WITH OTSC

The reported rate of complications after OTSC is very low. Most of these complications could have been avoided if a standardized approach was adopted. Review of literature has not yielded any specific pattern for occurrence of complications (**Table 1**).[7,12–26] To improve understanding, we have classified complications as those that occur (a) during the setup of the device, (b) during the clip deployment, and (c) during the endoscopic retrieval.

DURING DEVICE SETUP

The OTSC releases from the cap when a tension is exerted on the thread during setting up. Although the device assembly is similar to the band ligation system, there is no safety or auto-lock mechanism to prevent accidental release of the clip. During the hands-on training courses, we have observed participants accidently releasing the clip in the air or capturing their fingertips.[27] Similarly, attempting to remount the clip over the cap without the assistance of suitable accessories may result in injury to the fingers (**Fig. 4**).

Tips for Safety

We suggest fixing the cap onto the endoscope tip first before fastening the thread in the hand wheel. Always adjust the OTSC cap by pressing on the distal rim and not holding it by the sides. It prevents accidental dislodgement or loosening of the clip. The OTSC system is premounted with a clip. However, in situations whereby remounting needs to be performed, the approved reloading device should be used.

DURING OTSC INSERTION

The endoscopist must be aware that the OTSC cap is rigid with a thicker rim than the band ligation device. The outer diameter of the distal end of endoscope increases significantly after mounting with an OTSC. Hence, resistance can be encountered when advancing through acute bends, strictures, and narrower parts of the GI tract. Beginners usually find it difficult to navigate the OTSC mounted endoscope through the upper esophageal sphincter (UES). Any inadvertent and forceful advancement may result in mucosal injury or even esophageal perforation (**Fig. 5**). Honegger and colleagues[24] reported the occurrence of esophageal laceration when attempting to advance a large (14 mm) OTSC across the UES. Similarly, Voermans and colleagues[14] and Wedi and colleagues[7] described an instance of esophageal and sigmoid diverticular perforation during advancement of the endoscope (**Fig. 6**).

Tips for Safety

Choose the right clip size because using a larger clip and attempting to advance through a narrow area may result in adverse events. Always introduce and advance the scope under direct vision and stop if any resistance is felt. Consider using an overtube when difficulty is encountered at the UES.

DURING OTSC DEPLOYMENT

The complications that occur during OTSC deployment may be (a) technique related, (b) treatment related, and (c) underlying pathologic condition related.

Table 1
Complications with OTSC application

Author (y)	Cases with Complication	Type of Complication	Intervention
Albert et al,[12] 2011	Forrest 1b duodenal ulcer	GI leak	Surgical closure
Surace et al,[13] 2011	GI fistula	Anchor trapped in clip	Repeat endoscopy and anchor removal 7 d later
Voermans et al,[14] 2012	Duodenal perforation	Esophageal perforation during insertion	Thoracoscopic closure
Mangiavillano et al,[15] 2012	Duodenal perforation	Accidental released in tongue	Manual removal of clip
Baron et al,[16] 2012	Iatrogenic perforation Roux-en-Y anastomotic dehiscence Rectal fistula	Jejunal wall closure Gastrojejunostomy closure Pneumoperitoneum	Surgical closure Conservative treatment Conservative treatment
Hagel et al,[17] 2012	2.3-cm esophagojejunal anastomotic dehiscence Malignant perforation at posterior duodenal bulb	Enlargement of perforation Enlargement of perforation	Surgical closure Conservative treatment
Mercky et al,[18] 2015	Esophagogastric fistula after LSG Gastro-cutaneous fistula after LSG	Gastric stenosis Tearing of fistula edge with grasper	SEMS Conservative treatment
Rahmi et al,[19] 2015	Colonic perforation	Clipping of ureter	Surgical closure
Wedi et al,[7] 2016	Postcolonic EMR perforation closure Esophageal muscle injury after EMR	Sigmoid perforation during scope insertion Grasper trapped in clip	Surgical closure Mechanical dislodgement
Donatelli et al,[20] 2016	Leak following sleeve gastrectomy GI fistula	Stricture at gastroesophageal junction Migration of over the scope clip across fistula	SEMS Conservative treatment
Lokse et al,[21] 2016	Colonic perforation	Clipping of jejunum	Surgical removal
Raithel et al,[22] 2017	Duodenal perforation after colorectal resection Esophageal perforation after tumor resection Malignant perforation at posterior duodenal bulb Iatrogenic sigmoid perforation	Local peritonitis Enlargement of perforation ostium Peritonitis Small bowel fixation rupture	Conservative treatment Surgical closure Conservative treatment Surgical closure

(continued on next page)

Table 1 (continued)			
Author (y)	Cases with Complication	Type of Complication	Intervention
Kobara et al,[23] 2017	Post gastric ESD 5-cm perforation	Enlargement of perforation with misplaced clips	Surgical closure
Honegger et al,[24] 2017	Upper GI Esophageal anastomosis dehiscence Upper GI Lower GI	Accidental released in the tongue Increase in size of dehiscence Mucosal laceration in esophagus Rectal obstruction from pseudopolyp	Side cutter to remove Conservative treatment Conservative treatment
Khater et al,[25] 2017	Rectosigmoid perforation	Right ureter obstruction	Surgical removal
Tashima et al,[26] 2018	Duodena ESD perforation	Misplacement of clip caused expansion of defect	Closed with second OTSC

Abbreviations: EMR, endoscopic mucosal resection; ESD, endoscopic submucosal dissection; LSG, laparoscopic sleeve gastrectomy; SEMS, self-expandable metallic stent.

Technique Related

The success with OTSC is closely dependent on the precision of its deployment. Misplacement and superficial placement of OTSC occur when an adequate amount of tissue is not captured within the cap.[28] It may also result in accidental attachment of the OTSC accessories to the clip or the bowel wall (**Fig. 7**). Surace and colleagues[13] and Wedi and colleagues[7] reported capturing of OTSC anchor and

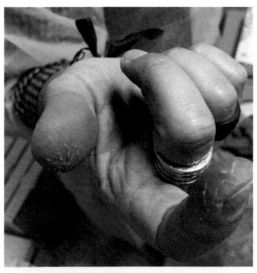

Fig. 4. Superficial injury at the fingertips while remounting the OTSC over the cap. The clip was accidently released on the finger, resulting in skin cuts.

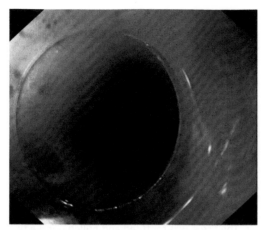

Fig. 5. Esophageal laceration with forceful advancement of the OTSC across the UES.

grasper within the teeth of the clip (see **Fig. 3**). In one of the cases, the anchor could not be removed immediately and was left in place. A repeat endoscopy was performed 7 days later to remove the anchor. Likewise, familiarity with accessory devices is necessary because improper use may result in mucosal injury or even perforation.

Treatment Related

Most serious complications reported so far with OTSC were treatment related. It is therefore vital to have an understanding of the nature of the lesion being treated; its relation to the surrounding structure, because OTSC can penetrate through the deeper layer of the bowel wall; and orientation of the endoscope to ensure accurate and safe clip placement.

Contained leak, pneumoperitoneum, and peritonitis have been described when deploying the OTSC and its accessories in thin-walled structures or excavated lesions (**Fig. 8**).[12,16] They were managed conservatively with a resolution of symptoms.

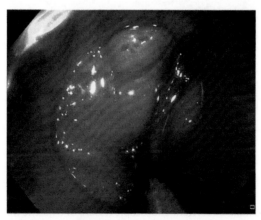

Fig. 6. Scope equipped with a medium-sized OTSC was advanced to treat a recurrent diverticular bleed. Perforation occurred when crossing an acute bend in the sigmoid colon.

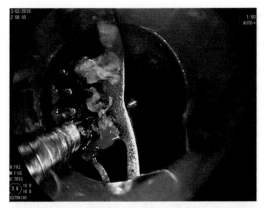

Fig. 7. Entrapment of an OTSC twin grasper within the clip. The OTSC was used to anchor a stent in the esophagus. The tissue was captured and pulled using a twin grasper. However, even before the twin grasper was sufficiently retracted, the clip was deployed and resulted in entrapment of the accessory.

However, serious complications requiring surgery for inadvertent capturing of the adjacent structure by OTSC have been reported. Loske and colleagues[21] and Raithel and colleagues[22] revealed small bowel fixation during treatment of colonic perforation using OTSC (**Fig. 9**). Similarly, Khater and colleagues[25] showed entrapment of right ureter causing obstruction while closing a sigmoid perforation with OTSC. In these cases, surgical repair and OTSC removal were required (**Fig. 10**). When treating perforation, there is a tendency to capture as much tissue as possible to achieve a complete tissue seal. However, this can also result in unintended inclusion of adjacent structures into the clip, causing complications.

Furthermore, occlusion of the GI lumen was described to occur when there is a loss of orientation during OTSC deployment. Baron and colleagues[16] showed 2 cases of inadvertent closure of opposing walls of jejunum with OTSC while treating an iatrogenic perforation and anastomotic dehiscence. Surgery was required in one to relieve

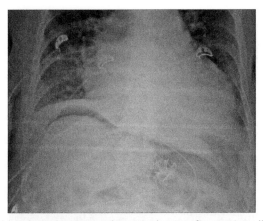

Fig. 8. A 75-year-old male underwent endoscopic closure of a gastric wall perforation using OTSC. Residual pneumoperitoneum was observed after successful clip closure. The patient remained asymptomatic after the procedure.

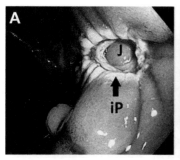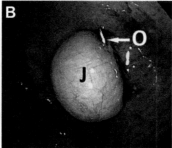

Fig. 9. Closure of an iatrogenic colonic perforation using an OTSC. (*A*) Iatrogenic transmural perforation defect (iP) of the colon after polypectomy. The small intestine (J) can be seen through the defect. (*B*) An attempt to close the perforation using an OTSC (O) resulted in the small intestine (J) being grasped by the clip. (*From* Loske, G., Schorsch, T., Daseking, E., Martens, E. and Müller, C. (2016) Small intestine grasped by over the scope clip during attempt to close an iatrogenic colonic perforation. Endoscopy 48: e26–e27.)

the obstruction. Similarly, Donatelli and colleagues and others[18,20] have illustrated the occurrence of gastric stenosis with OTSC during treatment of leak and esophagogastric fistula after laparoscopic sleeve gastrectomy, respectively (**Fig. 11**). Sometimes, the long retention time with OTSC may result in excessive hyperplastic polypoid-like tissue growth around the clip, which can cause luminal narrowing.[24] The tissue overgrowth and resultant narrowing can be managed successfully by endoscopy without requiring surgery.

Pathologic Condition Related

The success and complication rates associated with OTSC are also dependent on the type of lesion being treated. Of the different causes, the success rate is lower when managing a chronic fistula.[9] Similarly, the occurrence of complications may also be frequent when treating chronic, nonpliable, and unhealthy tissue, such as anastomotic dehiscence or fistula.

Donatelli and colleagues[20] presented a case of OTSC migration through the fistula orifice into the abdominal cavity. Raithel and colleagues and other investigators[18,22,26] showed enlargement of the size of perforation or dehiscence while treating using OTSC. Surgery remained the mainstay to address such unfavorable outcomes.

Tips for safety

We recommend adjusting the depth of the cap to the desired length when treating perforation. Using CO_2 insufflation during such treatment is prudent. We suggest not advancing the scope through the perforation ostia because it may enlarge the size of the defect. When only the suction method is applied to close a defect, rehearsing the maneuver before clip deployment may avoid inadvertent capturing of the adjacent structures. We encourage the use of accessories (Twin Grasper) for precisely capturing the right amount of tissue. The accessories must be sufficiently retracted inside the cap before clip deployment to prevent entrapment of accessories.

DURING ENDOSCOPE REMOVAL

The release of OTSC is seamless and smooth when the endoscope is straight and the lesion is in the en face view. One or 2 complete rotations of the hand wheel will release

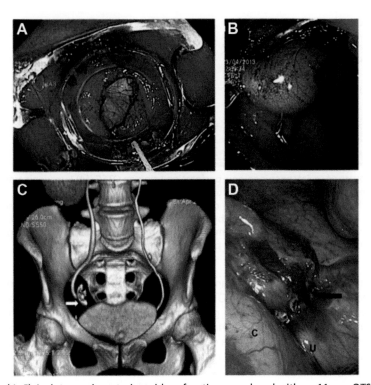

Fig. 10. (*A, B*) An iatrogenic rectosigmoid perforation was closed with an 11-mm OTSC using the twin grasper. (*C*) Follow-up computed tomographic scan to assess the perforation closure showed no leak but dilatation of the right ureter above the clip (arrow). (*D*) Because the clip could not be removed (arrow), the right ureter (U) was ligated at laparotomy, and a double-J catheter was placed. A short segment colon (c) resection was performed at the same time. The patient was discharged after 10 days without urinary symptoms. (*From* Rahmi G, Barret M, Samaha E, et al. Ureteral obstruction after colonoscopic perforation closed with an over-the-scope clip. Gastrointestinal Endoscopy. Volume 81, issue 2; 2015;470-72.)

the clip instantly. However, the OTSC deployment can be difficult when approaching the lesion tangentially in the esophagus and posterior duodenal wall or in a retroflexed position.[29] In a flexed endoscope position, the OTSC may sometimes fail to release despite multiple hand-wheel rotations. The clip continues to rest in the cap without capturing the target tissue, but upon straightening the scope, the clip dislodges suddenly from cap resulting in misplacement (**Fig. 12**).[15] Honegger and colleagues[24] reported 3 cases of accidental deployment of a large-sized OTSC in the tongue during endoscope withdrawal. A side cutter from an endoscopic retrograde cholangio-pancreatography tool kit was used to remove the misplaced clip.

Tips for Safety

We recommend maintaining a neutral and straight endoscope position where possible so that the axial force in the thread gets transmitted evenly and aids in smooth clip release. In difficult locations, we recommend using the accessories (OTSC anchor) to guide the OTSC. Last, confirm and photo-document clip deployment by visualizing the OTSC over the target site before withdrawing the scope.

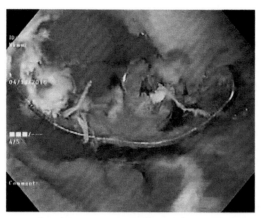

Fig. 11. Two OTSCs were placed to treat an esophageal fistula after Roux-en-Y esophagojejunostomy. Six weeks later, the patient presented with dysphagia and regurgitation. Endoscopy showed luminal obstruction at the level of the anastomosis. (*From* Rocha M, Küttner Magalhães R, Maia L, Moreira T, Barrias S, Nogueira C, Pedroto I: Endoscopic Removal of Two Esophageal Over-The-Scope Clips with Cold Saline Solution Technique. GE Port J Gastroenterol 2019;26:73-74. doi:10.1159/000487152; with permission.)

OTSC REMOVAL

OTSC once deployed can be difficult to remove and can interfere with subsequent therapy.[30] Thus, precise placement is crucial. Most clips detach and drop off spontaneously from the GI tract within months. However, some can stay longer, depending on the amount of tissue initially captured and the viability of the surrounding mucosa.

The OTSC is usually left in place because it is inert and causes no symptoms. Nonetheless, removal of OTSC may be required when (a) a complication occurs, (b) the clip

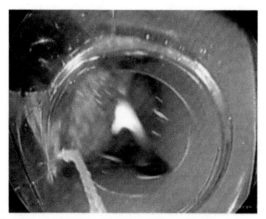

Fig. 12. Accidental release of OTSC in the tongue during insertion. (*From* Mangiavillano B, Morandi E, Masci E. Accidental endoscopic piercing of the tongue with an Ovesco clip. Endoscopy 2012; with permission.)

is misplaced, (c) removal of stent is fixed with OTSC, and (d) surveillance or resection of the residual lesion is required after full-thickness resection.

Several methods were described in the literature for OTSC removal with varying success rates.[31–33] Recently, a novel cutting device (remOVe system; Ovesco, Tubingen, Germany) has been made available to assist with OTSC removal. It consists of a bipolar grasping device with 3 distal electrodes and uses DC current to melt the nitinol clip. It is recommended to apply the DC impulse to the opposing hinges, the thinnest part of the OTSC, to dislodge the clip (**Fig. 13**). After displacement, the fragments can be safely removed using a forceps device. To avoid mucosal injury during extraction of clip fragments, We advise using a distal attachment cap. It is proposed that the thermal injury to the surrounding mucosa is only superficial and minimal and, in addition, the device is programmed to stop automatically when the electrodes are not in contact with nitinol. Bauder and colleagues[34] demonstrated that the remOVE system could be successfully used (97%) to fragment the OTSC in both the upper and the lower GI tract without complications.

ALTERNATIVE TECHNIQUES

Few other methods, like using argon plasma coagulation, Nd:YAG laser, endoscopic mucosal resection/endoscopic submucosal dissection resection of tissue at clip base, and guide wire–assisted removal, have been described in small case series.[31–33] The success rate with these methods can be variable, and there is a potential risk for excessive thermal injury. Of interest is the technique described by Arezzo and colleagues[33] whereby they used cold saline infusion for a minute to deform and remove

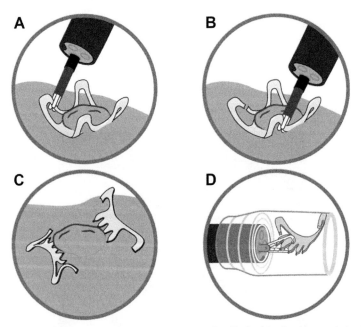

Fig. 13. Removal of OTSC using the remOVE system. (*A, B*) The bipolar electrode is placed at the hinge of OTSC. The DC current is applied, and the clip is fragmented. The fragments (*C*) are safely removed using a forceps by pulling it inside the cap (*D*). (*Courtesy of* Ovesco Endoscopy AG, Tubingen, Germany.)

the clip. They postulated that by reducing the temperature to less than 10° celcius, the grid structure of OTSC changes and makes it more malleable and allows easy removal with minimal resistance. Further reports are required to confirm the efficacy of this method.

SUMMARY

OTSC is a safe, effective, and important tool in the GI armamentarium for the treatment of GI bleeding, perforation, leak, and fistula. The overall complication rates reported to date with OTSC are extremely low and do not follow any specific pattern. Thus, the fear of complications should not limit its application in daily practice. The learning curve with OTSC is short. Understanding and mastering the device may help overcome most complications.

REFERENCES

1. Schecter WP, Hirshberg A, Chang DS, et al. Enteric fistulas: principles of management. J Am Coll Surg 2009;209:484–91.
2. Willingham FF, Buscaglia JM. Endoscopic management of gastrointestinal leaks and fistulae. Clin Gastroenterol Hepatol 2015;13(10):1714–21.
3. Available at: https://www.accessdata.fda.gov/cdrh_docs/pdf12/K120814.pdf. Accessed December 1, 2010.
4. Kirschniak A, Subotova N, Zieker D, et al. The over-the-scope clip for the treatment of gastrointestinal bleeding, perforations, and fistulas. Surg Endosc 2011; 25:2901–5.
5. Wedi E, Fischer A, Hochberger J, et al. Multicenter evaluation of first-line endoscopic treatment with the OTSC in acute non-variceal upper gastrointestinal bleeding and comparison with the Rockall cohort: the FLETRock study. Surg Endosc 2018;32(1):307–14.
6. Schmidt A, Gölder S, Goetz M, et al. Over-the-scope clips are more effective than standard endoscopic therapy for patients with recurrent bleeding of peptic ulcers. Gastroenterology 2018;155(3):674–86.e6.
7. Wedi E, Gonzalez S, Menke D, et al. One hundred and one over-the-scope-clip applications for severe gastrointestinal bleeding, leaks and fistulas. World J Gastroenterol 2016;22(5):1844–53.
8. Asokkumar R, Soetikno R, Sanchez-Yague A, et al. Use of over-the-scope-clip (OTSC) improves outcomes of high-risk adverse outcome (HR-AO) non-variceal upper gastrointestinal bleeding (NVUGIB). Endosc Int Open 2018;6(7):E789–96.
9. Kobara H, Mori H, Nishiyama N, et al. Over-the-scope clip system: a review of 1517 cases over 9 years. J Gastroenterol Hepatol 2019;34:22–30.
10. Schurr MO, Hartmann C, Ho CN, et al. An over-the-scope clip (OTSC) system for closure of iatrogenic colon perforations: results of an experimental survival study in pigs. Endoscopy 2008;40(7):584–8.
11. Asokkumar R, Kaltenbach T, Soetikno R. Use of over-the-scope clip to treat bleeding duodenal ulcers. Gastrointest Endosc 2016;83(2):459–60.
12. Albert JG, Friedrich-Rust M, Woeste G, et al. Benefit of a clipping device in use in intestinal bleeding and intestinal leakage. Gastrointest Endosc 2011;74(2): 389–97.
13. Surace M, Mercky P, Demarquay JF, et al. Endoscopic management of GI fistulae with the over-the-scope clip system (with video). Gastrointest Endosc 2011;74: 1416–9.

14. Voermans RP, Le Moine O, von Renteln D, et al. Efficacy of endoscopic closure of acute perforations of the gastrointestinal tract. Clin Gastroenterol Hepatol 2012; 10:603–8.
15. Mangiavillano B, Morandi E, Masci E. Accidental endoscopic piercing of the tongue with an Ovesco clip. Endoscopy 2012;44(Suppl 2 UCTN):E221.
16. Baron TH, Song LM, Ross A, et al. Use of an over-the-scope clipping device: multicenter retrospective results of the first U.S. experience (with videos). Gastrointest Endosc 2012;76:202–8.
17. Hagel AF, Naegel A, Lindner AS, et al. Over-the-scope clip application yields a high rate of closure in gastrointestinal perforations and may reduce emergency surgery. J Gastrointest Surg 2012;16:2132–8.
18. Mercky P, Gonzalez JM, Aimore Bonin E, et al. Usefulness of over-the scope clipping system for closing digestive fistulas. Dig Endosc 2015;27:18–24.
19. Rahmi G, Barret M, Samaha E, et al. Ureteral obstruction after colonoscopic perforation closed with an over-the-scope clip. Gastrointest Endosc 2015;81(2): 470–1.
20. Donatelli G, Cereatti F, Dhumane P, et al. Closure of gastrointestinal defects with Ovesco clip: long-term results and clinical implications. Therap Adv Gastroenterol 2016;9:713–21.
21. Loske G, Schorsch T, Daseking E, et al. Small intestine grasped by over-the-scope-clip during attempt to close an iatrogenic colonic perforation. Endoscopy 2016;48:e26–7.
22. Raithel M, Albrecht H, Scheppach W, et al. Outcome, comorbidity, hospitalization and 30-day mortality after closure of acute perforations and postoperative anastomotic leaks by the over-the-scope clip (OTSC) in an unselected cohort of patients. Surg Endosc 2017;31:2411–25.
23. Kobara H, Mori H, Fujihara S, et al. Outcomes of gastrointestinal defect closure with an over-the-scope clip system in a multicenter experience: An analysis of a successful suction method. World J Gastroenterol 2017;23(9): 1645–56.
24. Honegger C, Valli PV, Wiegand N, et al. Establishment of over-the-scope-clips (OTSC®) in daily endoscopic routine. United Eur Gastroenterol J 2017;5: 247–54.
25. Khater S, Rahmi G, Perrod G, et al. Over-the-scope clip (OTSC) reduces surgery rate in the management of iatrogenic gastrointestinal perforations. Endosc Int Open 2017;5:E389–94.
26. Tashima T, Ohata K, Sakai E, et al. Efficacy of an over-the-scope clip for preventing adverse events after duodenal endoscopic submucosal dissection: a prospective interventional study. Endoscopy 2018;50:487–96.
27. Soetikno R, Asokkumar R, Salazar E, et al. Flipped learning in endoscopy: a time effective model to impacr change in practice culture. Gastrointest Endosc 2019; 89(6):AB410–1.
28. Asokkumar R, Sanchez-Yague A, Soetikno R. Incomplete hemostasis of high-risk adverse outcome bleeding lesions after placement of the over-the-scope clip: causes and solutions. VideoGIE 2018;3(5):155–6.
29. Chan SM, Lau JY. Can we now recommend OTSC as first-line therapy in case of non-variceal upper gastrointestinal bleeding? Endosc Int Open 2017;5(9): E883–5.
30. Asokkumar R, Soetikno R. Misplaced "bear claw" in a bleeding gastric ulcer: what next? Gastrointest Endosc 2016;84(2):366–7.

31. Fähndrich M, Sandmann M, Heike M. Removal of over the scope clips (OTSC) with an Nd:YAG Laser. Z Gastroenterol 2011;49:579–83.
32. Neumann H, Diebel H, Monkemuller K, et al. Description of a new, endoscopic technique to remove the over-the-scope-clip in an ex vivo porcine model (with video). Gastrointest Endosc 2012;76:1009–13.
33. Arezzo A, Bullano A, Fischer H, et al. The way to remove an over-the-scope-clip (with video). Gastrointest Endosc 2013;77(6):974–5.
34. Bauder M, Meier B, Caca K, et al. Endoscopic removal of over-the-scope clips: clinical experience with a bipolar cutting device. United Eur Gastroenterol J 2017;5(4):479–84.

Clipping Over the Scope for Recurrent Peptic Ulcer Bleeding is Cost-Effective as Compared to Standard Therapy: An Initial Assessment

Jessica X. Yu, MD, MS[a],*, W. Alton Russell, MS[b],
Ravishankar Asokkumar, MBBS, MD, MRCP[c],
Tonya Kaltenbach, MD, MS[d,e,f],
Roy Soetikno, MD, MS (Health Services Research), MS (Management)[f]

KEYWORDS

- Peptic ulcer disease • Clipping over the scope • Clipping through the scope
- Thermal devices

KEY POINTS

- For second-line therapy, repeating standard therapy (ST) after failed ST is not cost-effective.
- For first-line therapy, clipping over the scope (C-OTS) may be considered for patients with intermediate- or high-risk ulcers as determined by the Rockall score.
- Further cost-effectiveness analyses of C-OTS compared with ST requires additional studies on the effectiveness of C-OTS compared with ST.

INTRODUCTION

Peptic ulcer disease (PUD) is the most common cause of nonvariceal upper gastro-intestinal bleeding and is associated with mortality rates of up to 10%.[1] Standard endoscopic therapy with thermal and mechanical interventions is highly effective although the rates of rebleeding range from 8% to 15%.[2] For certain lesions that

[a] Division of Gastroenterology and Hepatology, University of Michigan, 1301 Catherine Street, Ann Arbor, MI 48109, USA; [b] Department of Management Sciences and Engineering, Stanford University, 475 Via Ortega, Stanford, CA 94305, USA; [c] Department of Gastroenterology and Hepatology, Singapore General Hospital, Outram Road, Singapore 169608, Singapore; [d] Division of Gastroenterology and Hepatology, University of California San Francisco, 513 Parnassus Avenue, San Francisco, CA 94143, USA; [e] Department of Gastroenterology, Veterans Affairs Medical Center; [f] Advanced Gastrointestinal Endoscopy, Mountain View, CA, USA
* Corresponding author. Division of Gastroenterology and Hepatology, Oregon Health and Sciences University, 3181 Southwest Sam Jackson Park Road, Mail Code: L461, Portland, OR 97239.
E-mail address: yujess@ohsu.edu

Gastrointest Endoscopy Clin N Am 30 (2020) 91–97
https://doi.org/10.1016/j.giec.2019.09.004
1052-5157/20/© 2019 Elsevier Inc. All rights reserved.

are at high risk for adverse outcomes, such as those with large-caliber visible vessels and fibrotic ulcers with high-risk stigmata, the rates of rebleeding may be 40%.[3] Clipping over the scope (C-OTS) is a novel closure technique used for the treatment of nonvariceal gastrointestinal bleeding, especially for high-risk lesions. Compared with standard clipping through the scope (C-TTS), C-OTS allows for high-pressure closure of larger mucosal areas and deeper layers. A recent randomized controlled trial demonstrated lower rebleeding with C-OTS using Ovesco (Ovesco AG, Tubingen, Germany) compared with standard therapy (ST) with C-TTS or thermal therapy for persistent or recurrent PUD bleeding.[4] However, C-OTS costs more than C-TTS and thermal devices. The high upfront cost of C-OTS may pose a barrier to its use and the cost-effectiveness of C-OTS for PUD bleeding is unknown.

We sought to determine the cost-effectiveness of using C-OTS for peptic ulcer bleeding as both first-line and second-line therapy. We aimed to identify the cost and effectiveness of C-OTS for PUD bleeding as compared with ST use as either first-line or second-line therapy. We hypothesized that despite the higher cost, C-OTS, with its lower risk of persistent/recurrent bleeding, is cost-effective to use in the first-line and second-line management of PUD bleeding.

METHODS
Model Design

We used a decision tree to model the cost, effectiveness, and rates of persistent/recurrent bleeding from C-OTS versus ST for the treatment of a patient with peptic ulcer bleeding over a 30-day time horizon (**Fig. 1**). We compared the cost-effectiveness of the modalities by calculating the incremental cost-effectiveness ratio. We considered a strategy to be cost-effective if it was lower than the willing-to-pay threshold of $100,000 per quality-adjusted life year (QALY).

We modeled three possible treatment strategies for a patient admitted with PUD bleeding. In the first treatment strategy (ST/C-OTS), the patient has an esophagogastroduodenoscopy (EGD) with ST as the first-line therapy. If the first-line ST results in persistent/recurrent bleeding, then a second EGD with C-OTS is performed as the second-line therapy. If the second-line therapy remains unsuccessful, then we assumed the patient underwent interventional radiology (IR) or surgery. In the second

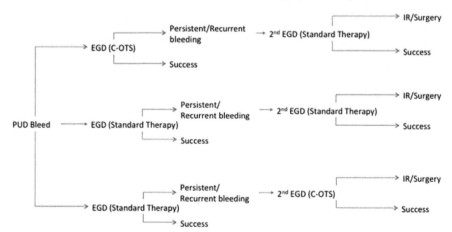

Fig. 1. Decision tree to model costs, effectiveness (quality-adjusted life years), and rates of persistent/recurrent bleeding of C-OTS versus standard therapy for the treatment of PUD bleeding. EGD, esophagogastroduodenoscopy; IR, interventional radiology.

treatment strategy (C-OTS/ST), an EGD with C-OTS is the first-line therapy. In this strategy, if the first-line therapy C-OTS was unsuccessful, then EGD with ST was used for second-line therapy because it is technically challenging to place a second C-OTS device after initial C-OTS. Finally, we assessed the third treatment strategy (ST/ST), which started with EGD with ST as the first-line therapy. In this strategy, if ST resulted in persistent/recurrent bleeding, then a repeat EGD with ST as the second-line therapy was performed. For all three treatment strategies, if the second-line treatment strategy is unsuccessful, we assume that the patient then proceeds with IR or surgery. These were assumed to be successful.

Base Case Model Inputs

Model inputs are summarized in **Table 1**. The costs of the devices were based on costs from the US Veterans Administration healthcare system. Cost of C-OTS was based on the Ovesco clip. Cost of an ST was based on a mean of the cost of a C-TTS (Resolution 360, Boston Scientific, Marlborough, MA) and the cost of a Gold Probe (Boston Scientific). The cost of an EGD for hemostasis (Current Procedural Terminology code 43255) and hospitalization were estimated (MS DRG 379, 377, 378) from 2016 Centers for Medicare and Medicaid data.

The probability of persistent/recurrent bleeding with C-OTS and ST as the first-line therapy was obtained through review of the literature on the use of standard clip/thermal therapy and the use of Ovesco clips on PUD bleeding published

Table 1
Summary of key model inputs for our base case analysis

	C-OTS	Standard Therapy
Initial cost of PUD bleeding (cost of device + cost of EGD + hospitalization)	$6165 ($438 + $193 + 5534)	$5901 ($174 + 193 + 5534)
Cost of PUD with persistent/ recurrent bleeding treated endoscopically	$8766	$8238
Cost of PUD with persistent/ recurrent bleeding requiring IR/surgery	$15,365	$14,836
Probability of persistent/ recurrent bleeding, first-line therapy	0.05	0.11
Probability of IR/surgery, second-line therapy	0.15	0.58
Initial utility loss of PUD bleeding	−0.013	−0.013
Utility loss, PUD with persistent/recurrent bleeding treated endoscopically	−0.016	−0.016
Utility loss, PUD requiring IR/surgery	−0.026	−0.026

Costs of devices are from the Veterans Administration system and costs of the hospitalization and procedure were estimated from Centers for Medicare and Medicaid 2016 data. Probability of persistent/recurrent bleeding for C-OTS with Ovesco clips as first-line therapy derived from literature review.[5–8] The probability of persistent/recurrent bleeding from standard therapy as first-line therapy is also derived from literature review.[9–16] Utilities were estimated from literature.[17]

between 2014 and 2019.[5–16] For C-OTS as first-line therapy, studies in which C-OTS was used for nonvariceal upper gastrointestinal bleeding were included if PUD represented most cases. Only outcomes of C-OTS and ST as first-line therapy were included. The probability of needing IR or surgery after a failed second-line endoscopic therapy with C-OTS or ST was obtained from the recently published STING randomized control trial.[4] Utility losses were also obtained for literature review.[17] Given the short time horizon of our study, we assumed there was no mortality.

Sensitivity Analyses

We performed one-way sensitivity analyses on all variables. To determine if C-OTS would be preferred as first-line therapy, we performed two-way sensitivity analyses on rates of persistent/recurrent bleeding with C-OTS versus rates of persistent/recurrent bleeding with ST. We compared the specific scenarios of treating medium-risk (Rockall score 4–7) and high-risk ulcers (Rockall score >7) and estimated the risk of persistent/recurrent bleeding from Wedi and colleagues[8]

RESULTS
Base Case

We found that the first treatment strategy of ST for first-line therapy followed by C-OTS as second-line therapy was the most cost-effective strategy, costing $6298 per patient and resulting in 0.0686 QALYs (**Fig. 2**). This was associated with an 11% rate of persistent/recurrent bleeding after a failed first-line therapy and a 1.7% rate of requiring IR/surgery after a failed second-line therapy. Using C-OTS as first-line with ST as second-line cost $6490 and 0.0687 QALYs, but was not cost-effective compared with ST/C-OTS with an incremental cost-effectiveness ratio of $5,858,937. The third treatment strategy of ST followed by ST cost $6576 and resulted in 0.0659 QALYs. Therefore, this strategy is not cost-effective.

Sensitivity Analysis

Our model was sensitive to the cost of C-OTS and ST, cost of hospitalization of persistent/recurrent bleeding, and probability of persistent/recurrent bleeding with C-OTS. We found that the strategy of ST/C-OTS is not preferred if the cost of ST is greater than $378. In addition, the cost of C-OTS needed to fall lower than $221 for ST/C-OTS to no longer be preferred. The probability of requiring IR or surgery, for failed second-line C-OTS, needed to be greater than 0.38 and the probability of a failed second-line ST needed to fall below than 0.11.

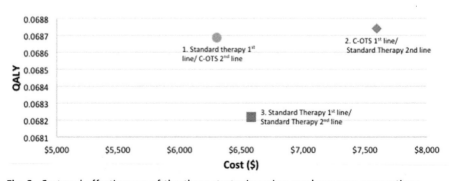

Fig. 2. Cost and effectiveness of the three strategies using our base case assumptions.

As the probability of persistent/recurrent bleeding following ST increases, C-OTS/ST becomes preferred in more scenarios (**Fig. 3**). Specifically, for medium- or high-risk ulcer with Rockall score greater than or equal to 4, then C-OTS as the first-line therapy followed by ST as second-line is preferred.

DISCUSSIONS

Our study found that the treatment strategy of EGD with ST as first-line therapy followed by EGD with C-OTS using Ovesco clips as second-line therapy for persistent/recurrent bleeding is the most cost-effective strategy when compared with ST as first-line therapy followed ST as second-line therapy and C-OTS as first-line therapy followed by ST as second-line therapy. Importantly, our model was sensitive to the cost of C-OTS and ST. In our base case, we used a cost of $174, which is the average cost of one C-TTS and the gold probe. However, in practice, more than one C-TTS may be placed, which may make ST as first-line no longer cost-effective.

C-OTS has been found to be more effective for persistent/refractory bleeding compared with ST and safe and effective for bleeding from HR-AO lesions. Herein, we included the cost to evaluate the cost-effectiveness. By varying the rate of persistent/recurrent bleeding with C-OTS versus ST as first-line, we found that C-OTS becomes preferred as first-line therapy if the rates of persistent/recurrent bleeding with ST increases. In our scenario analysis, we found that C-OTS is preferred as first-line therapy for medium- and high-risk peptic ulcer with Rockall scores greater than or equal to 4.

The use of sensitivity analyses gives insight into uncertainty in the model. We found that there are three other conditions that are determinants to the cost-effectiveness of C-OTS: (1) cost of C-OTS, (2) cost of the ST, and (3) the cost of hospitalization. In our analysis, we used the costs that are applicable to our own settings. Readers are suggested to consider their own settings and outcomes when using the results of this study.

There were a few limitations of our study. Our model inputs were largely based on observational studies, especially for EGD with C-OTS as the first-line therapy. Specifically, a randomized controlled trial comparing ST with C-OTS as the first-line therapy is still ongoing. There were also limited data on long-term outcomes and mortality on which to base our model. Further studies are still required to address these areas of uncertainty.

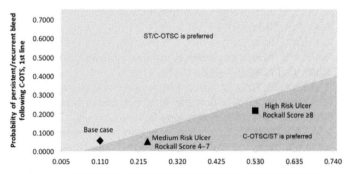

Fig. 3. Two-way sensitivity analysis when both the probability of persistent/recurrent bleeding after first-line C-OTS versus probability of persistent/recurrent bleeding after first standard therapy is varied.

In conclusion, for second-line therapy, repeating ST after failed ST is not cost-effective. Instead, C-OTS should be used for persistent/recurrent bleeding after failed ST. For first-line therapy, C-OTS may be considered for patients with intermediate- or high-risk ulcers as determined by the Rockall score. Additional studies on the effectiveness of C-OTS compared with ST for first-line therapy are needed to improve future cost-effectiveness evaluations.

ACKNOWLEDGMENTS

Presented as an oral presentation at the Digestive Disease Week, 2019.

REFERENCES

1. Laine L, McQuaid KR. Endoscopic therapy for bleeding ulcers: an evidence-based approach based on meta-analyses of randomized controlled trials. Clin Gastroenterol Hepatol 2009;7:33–47 [quiz: 1–2].
2. Lau JY, Barkun A, Fan DM, et al. Challenges in the management of acute peptic ulcer bleeding. Lancet 2013;381:2033–43.
3. Brandler J, Baruah A, Zeb M, et al. Efficacy of over-the-scope clips in management of high-risk gastrointestinal bleeding. Clin Gastroenterol Hepatol 2018; 16:690–6.e1.
4. Schmidt A, Golder S, Goetz M, et al. Over-the-scope clips are more effective than standard endoscopic therapy for patients with recurrent bleeding of peptic ulcers. Gastroenterology 2018;155:674–86.e6.
5. Manta R, Mangiafico S, Zullo A, et al. First-line endoscopic treatment with over-the-scope clips in patients with either upper or lower gastrointestinal bleeding: a multicenter study. Endosc Int Open 2018;6:E1317–21.
6. Asokkumar R, Soetikno R, Sanchez-Yague A, et al. Use of over-the-scope-clip (OTSC) improves outcomes of high-risk adverse outcome (HR-AO) non-variceal upper gastrointestinal bleeding (NVUGIB). Endosc Int Open 2018;6: E789–96.
7. Manno M, Mangiafico S, Caruso A, et al. First-line endoscopic treatment with OTSC in patients with high-risk non-variceal upper gastrointestinal bleeding: preliminary experience in 40 cases. Surg Endosc 2016;30:2026–9.
8. Wedi E, Fischer A, Hochberger J, et al. Multicenter evaluation of first-line endoscopic treatment with the OTSC in acute non-variceal upper gastrointestinal bleeding and comparison with the Rockall cohort: the FLETRock study. Surg Endosc 2018;32:307–14.
9. Kim JS, Kim BW, Park SM, et al. Factors associated with rebleeding in patients with peptic ulcer bleeding: analysis of the Korean peptic ulcer bleeding (K-PUB) study. Gut Liver 2018;12:271–7.
10. Chiu PWY, Joeng HK, Choi CL, et al. High-dose omeprazole infusion compared with scheduled second-look endoscopy for prevention of peptic ulcer rebleeding: a randomized controlled trial. Endoscopy 2016;48:717–22.
11. Lu Y, Barkun AN, Martel M. Adherence to guidelines: a national audit of the management of acute upper gastrointestinal bleeding. The REASON registry. Can J Gastroenterol Hepatol 2014;28:495–501.
12. Vergara M, Bennett C, Calvet X, et al. Epinephrine injection versus epinephrine injection and a second endoscopic method in high-risk bleeding ulcers. Cochrane Database Syst Rev 2014:CD005584. https://doi.org/10.1002/14651858. CD005584.pub3.

13. Lanas A, Carrera-Lasfuentes P, Garcia-Rodriguez LA, et al. Outcomes of peptic ulcer bleeding following treatment with proton pump inhibitors in routine clinical practice: 935 patients with high- or low-risk stigmata. Scand J Gastroenterol 2014;49:1181–90.

14. Sung JJY, Suen BY, Wu JCY, et al. Effects of intravenous and oral esomeprazole in the prevention of recurrent bleeding from peptic ulcers after endoscopic therapy. Am J Gastroenterol 2014;109:1005–10.

15. Marmo R, Koch M, Cipolletta L, et al. Predicting mortality in patients with in-hospital nonvariceal upper GI bleeding: a prospective, multicenter database study. Gastrointest Endosc 2014;79:741–9.e1.

16. de Groot NL, van Oijen MG, Kessels K, et al. Reassessment of the predictive value of the Forrest classification for peptic ulcer rebleeding and mortality: can classification be simplified? Endoscopy 2014;46:46–52.

17. Speigel BMR, Dulai GS, Lims BS, et al. The Cost-Effectiveness and Budget Impact of Intravenous Versus Oral Proton Pump Inhibitors in Peptic Ulcer Hemorrhage. Clin Gastroenterol Hepatol 2006;4:988–97.

Rapid and Safe Crossing of the Chasm

Application of a Flipped Learning Framework for the Clipping Over the Scope Technique

Roy Soetikno, MD, MS (Health Services Research), MS (Management)[a,*],
Ravishankar Asokkumar, MBBS, MD, MRCP[b],
Yung-Ka Chin, MD, MBChB, MRCP[b], Ennaliza Salazar, MD[b],
Tiffany Nguyen-Vu, BA[c], Silvia Sanduleanu, MD, PhD[d],
Jason Chang Pik Eu, MD[b], Tonya Kaltenbach, MD, MS[a,c,e]

KEYWORDS

- Clipping over the scope • Flipped learning framework • Gastrointestinal bleeding
- Endoscopic balloon dilation

KEY POINTS

- Users of high-tech medical devices can be classified into at least 5 different categories: innovators, early adopters, early majority, late majority, and laggards. New technology does not flow independently from 1 group of users to the next.
- Gaps exist between the different kinds of users and may prevent the downstream movement of technology. The largest gap, known as "the chasm," lies between the early adopters and the early majority users.
- The flipped learning pedagogy is a commonly used learning model in higher education. In flipped learning, the traditional classroom environment is reversed by predelivering the instructional material before the class through the learning management system and the classroom is used for experiential hands-on training using biorealistic models.

Continued

Disclosure Statement: Dr R. Soetikno is a consultant for Olympus America. Dr T. Kaltenbach is a consultant for Olympus America and Aries Pharmaceuticals. Dr R. Asokkumar, Dr Y.K. Chin, Dr E. Salazar, Dr J. Chang Pik Eu, Dr S. Sanduleanu, and Ms T. Nguyen-Vu have nothing to disclose.
[a] Advanced Gastrointestinal Endoscopy, Mountain View, CA, USA; [b] Department of Gastroenterology and Hepatology, Singapore General Hospital, Singapore; [c] Department of Gastroenterology, San Francisco Veterans Affairs Medical Center, San Francisco, CA, USA; [d] Division of Gastroenterology and Hepatology, Maastricht University Medical Center, Maastricht, the Netherlands; [e] Division of Gastroenterology and Hepatology, University of California San Francisco, San Francisco, CA, USA
* Corresponding author.
E-mail address: soetikno@earthlink.net

Gastrointest Endoscopy Clin N Am 30 (2020) 99–106
https://doi.org/10.1016/j.giec.2019.09.002
1052-5157/20/© 2019 Elsevier Inc. All rights reserved.

Continued

- We applied flipped learning to train and encourage a cohort of practicing gastroenterologists and fellows to adopt a relatively complex procedure, clipping over the scope, and an established yet underutilized technique, endoscopic balloon dilation, within a short time period.
- Using flipped learning appears beneficial for crossing the chasm in the adoption of high-tech medical devices.
- The clipping techniques include over the scope and through the scope, which can be abbreviated C-OTS and C-TTS, respectively.[a]

INTRODUCTION

For high-tech medical devices, which over the scope (OTS) clipping technologies could be classified as, Geoffrey A. Moore's theory of "Crossing the Chasm" provides a fundamental understanding of how users (gastroenterologists) adapt to new technologies. Moore shows that users can be classified into at least 5 different kinds: innovators, early adopters, early majority, late majority, and laggards. Furthermore, he demonstrates that there are gaps that may prevent the downstream movement of technology; technology does not independently flow from 1 kind of user to the next.[1] In particular, the most significant gap is the one between early adopters and early majority (**Fig. 1**). If this chasm is not crossed, the technology does not become mainstream.

In order to understand the gaps, the characteristics of the different groups of users will need to be analyzed (the different group of gastroenterologists). The innovators always seek out novel technology. They are willing to be on the cutting edge and always want to be the first to try new technology. The early adopters are different from the innovators. Although they do not love new technologies just for the same reasons, they are quick to grasp the potential benefits of emerging technology and its potential for new and strategic opportunities. The early majority, which accounts for most users (most gastroenterologists), are practical minded and cautious.[1,2] They are more concerned about data: quality, reliability, and support. They are more likely to communicate with others like themselves than with early adopters or innovators. An essential characteristic of the early majority is that they do not use the product until it is already established. However, the product would not get established unless they use it.

Based on our experience in our unit, we observed that clipping over the scope (C-OTS) for the treatment of high-risk and recurrent upper gastrointestinal bleeding (UGIB) was not adapted beyond a few gastroenterologists, who were most likely the early adopters. In order to cross the chasm, we conducted a department-wide course to train their gastroenterologists on the technique of C-OTS. Perhaps by enabling the early majority to learn about the indications and outcomes data and by giving them the opportunity to experience its deployment firsthand, they would be encouraged to adopt the device into their regular practice.

We designed the course using flipped learning, a pedagogical approach in which instructional cognitive content is delivered to the individual instead of the group, usually through online platforms and outside of the classroom, and experiential content to

---

[a] Note that the abbreviation for Over-The-Scope-Clips is trademarked and thus cannot be used to denote the technique of clipping using devices that are placed from outside of the endoscope.

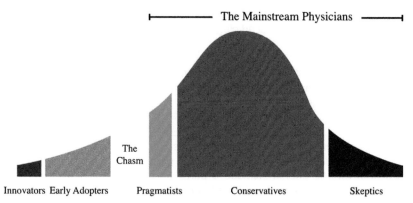

Fig. 1. The biggest gap exists between the early adapters and the early majority. (*Data from* Moore G. *Crossing the Chasm*. 3rd ed. New York, NY: Harper Business Essentials; 2014.)

learn the skills is provided in small groups in the classroom (**Fig. 2**). We trained the gastroenterologists on the technical skills required for simulators of C-OTS technique. Although flipped learning is commonly used and has been proven to be effective in higher education, including in medical schools, it is still infrequently used in endoscopy.[3,4] Herein, we describe our methods and results of the training courses on the techniques of C-OTS for gastrointestinal bleeding and endoscopic balloon dilation. We believe that our work is relevant because the adoption of new technology in gastroenterology is typically slow, and the chasms can be wide and deep.

METHODS

We conducted a prospective study at Singapore General Hospital between July 2018 and September 2018. We invited general gastroenterologists and fellows to participate in this novel modular training program. A waiver was obtained from the

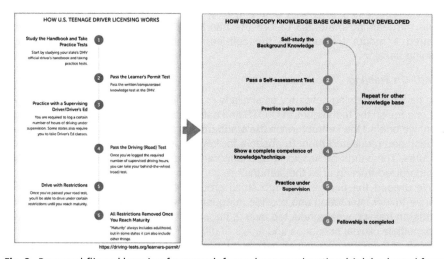

Fig. 2. Proposed flipped learning framework for endoscopy education (*right*) adapted from the learning paradigm of US teenage drivers' licensing (*left*).

Institutional Review Board for this study. All authors had access to the study data and reviewed and approved the final article.

Participants

We invited general gastroenterologists with varied duration of clinical experience and fellows in training to participate in the program. These participants were naive to the contents of the training program.

Course Design

The course was designed to train practicing gastroenterologists in a new technique, C-OTS to treat UGIB, and to train the fellows to perform balloon dilation through the scope (BD-TTS). The course included 3 parts: (a) precourse essential reading, (b) hands-on training on models, and (c) a brief lectures on the dos and don'ts of the C-OTS technique in the treatment of UGIB, lower gastrointestinal bleeding, and perforation.

We employed the flipped learning pedagogy and a cloud-based learning management system (LMS) to deliver the course content. With flipped learning, we reversed the traditional classroom environment by predelivering the instructional material before the class through their LMS. We used the classroom for experiential hands-on training using the biorealistic models.

Course Materials

We created multiple self-learning modules within the LMS to provide a cognitive knowledge base for the C-OTS and BD-TTS techniques. The materials included multiple instructional videos, seminal papers, procedural movies, and self-assessment questionnaires. The participants were required to complete the self-assessment quiz satisfactorily (scores >80%) before they could progress to the next module. The quizzes were derived from the course content and were structured to fulfill the Accreditation Council for Graduate Medical Education-I academic curriculum on the treatment of UGIB and esophageal dilation.[5] We allowed 3 attempts to complete the self-assessment questionnaire and did not provide the correct answers after each attempt. We monitored the progress and the performance of the participants periodically and delivered reminders at regular intervals to complete the learning materials before the hands-on training. The participants were allotted 1 month to complete the self-learning materials before the hands-on training session.

Hands-On Training

The hands-on training session was similarly extensive. The instructors had extensive experience on the techniques of C-OTS and balloon dilation. Before the hands-on session, we briefed the instructors on the standardized approach for C-OTS and balloon dilation and requested them to observe for key steps required to perform these procedures. The hands-on session was monitored by a moderator to ensure delivery of standardized training in all the stations.

We divided the participants into small groups (4 per station) to promote ample trainee-trainer interaction and provide adequate time for practice in the models. The hands-on training was conducted over 2.5 hours so that the participants could practice multiple clinical scenarios and levels of difficulty. There was no restriction on the number of C-OTS devices used per person or the number of dilations performed. We used the Ovesco Bleeding Model (Ovesco, Tubiegen, Germany) and the EMS Trainer (Chamberlain Group, Great Barrington, MA, USA) to train the C-OTS and BD-TTS, respectively. In addition, we used explant porcine models to simulate clinical experience and train the C-OTS technique on tissue.

We used the Ovesco Bleeding Model (Ovesco), which had simulated bleeding ulcers in different parts of the stomach and duodenum. They required the participants to deploy OTS clips on the ulcers that were easily accessible and on those situated in complex locations (high lesser curve and posterior duodenal wall). We assured that the process was based on deliberative practice and competency. Participants were given constructive feedback throughout the session until they became competent. We used a checklist to assure that the participants performed the procedure in a complete and step-by-step fashion.

We taught the participants the use of an Anchor, a triprong device that was made of nitinol and designed for anchoring and positioning fibrotic bleeding ulcers inside the cap of the OTS clipping device. After they were familiarized with the Anchor device, we introduced the application of the twin grasper. They created a 1-cm perforation in the explant porcine models and trained them to use the twin grasper to approximate the edges of perforation and seal it using an OTS clip. Throughout the course, the participants alternated the role of assistant and endoscopist to become familiar with all aspects of the procedural technique.

Data Collection

We collected information about the participants' level of training, experience, and their area of interest in Gastroenterology. We recorded the time spent by each participant in the LMS module before the hands-on training. We collected their scores on the self-assessment questionnaires after each module. We administered a brief anonymous survey to measure satisfactory outcomes for the course across a variety of domains using a 5-point Likert scale.

Outcomes Assessments

We evaluated the impact of the training program by collating data on the use of the C-OTS and BD-TTS techniques in real-world practice. We created a registry to track the number of such procedures performed within 4 months after the course. We captured the procedurist information, indication for treatment, technical success, and outcomes.

RESULTS
Characteristics of the Participants

We enrolled a total of 36 participants: 24 general gastroenterologists and 12 gastroenterology fellows. The majority were men (n = 30, 83.3%) with a mean age of 40 ± 10 years. All the gastroenterologists (mean duration of practice, 4.9 ± 4 years) completed the C-OTS course. Nine of them completed the BD-TTS course in addition. All the fellows (mean duration of training, 1.9 ± 1.6 years) completed both courses. The details of the participants are shown in **Table 1**.

Clipping Over the Scope

Most of the participants (69.4%, n = 25) reported no prior experience with C-OTS technique. Some participants (30.6%, n = 10) had limited prior experience (<5 clips), whereas one had significant experience (2.8%). A mean time of 1.4 ± 1.5 hours was spent on self-learning the cognitive material and 1.5 hours to practice the technical skills using the silicone and explant porcine models. Four months after the course, there was a 7-fold increase in the adoption rate of the C-OTS technique among

Table 1 Participant demographics (N = 36)	
Average age (range)	
40 (29–77)	
Gender (n, %)	
Male	30 (83.3)
Female	6 (16.7)
Experience level (n, %)	
General gastroenterologist	24 (66.7)
Gastrointestinal (GI) Fellow	12 (33.3)
Time in practice or in fellowship (y)	
General gastroenterologist	4.9 ± 4
GI Fellow	1.9 ± 1.6
Course enrollment (n, %)	
C-OTS	36 (100)
Dilation	21 (58.3)

gastroenterologists with no or minimal prior experience (22.2% vs 2.8%). OTS clips were successfully applied in 15 patients to treat bleeding (n = 11) and perforation (n = 4).

Dilation

Most of the participants (90.5%, n = 19) had no clinical experience with balloon dilation before the course. They spent 0.3 ± 0.2 hours to complete the self-learning and 1.5 hours for the experiential session. On follow-up 4 months after the course, there was a 3-fold increase in adoption rate for endoscopic balloon dilation among participants (28.6% vs 9.5%). Dilations were successfully performed in 9 patients to treat benign gastroesophageal strictures.

There were no complications observed with the above procedures.

Satisfaction

Of the 23 respondents, more than 91% strongly agreed or agreed that the course covered all the necessary materials in a reasonable amount of time. Ninety-six percent strongly agreed or agreed that the method for delivering the learning content was appropriate. All of the respondents (100%) indicated that they would participate in a similarly structured course for new topics in the future, with 78% indicating that they would be willing to pay for such courses (**Fig. 3**). A majority (n = 17) of the participants expressed the usefulness of the hands-on sessions by noting that the instructors were helpful, the models were realistic, and the hands-on experience helped to prepare them for clinical practice.

DISCUSSION

We demonstrated the efficacy of flipped learning in encouraging early majority gastroenterologists to use the C-OTS technique, a new innovation in the treatment of UGIB. We found that such an experience can facilitate the adoption of technology into clinical practice, enabling us to bring novel technologies to the early majority, crossing the chasm.

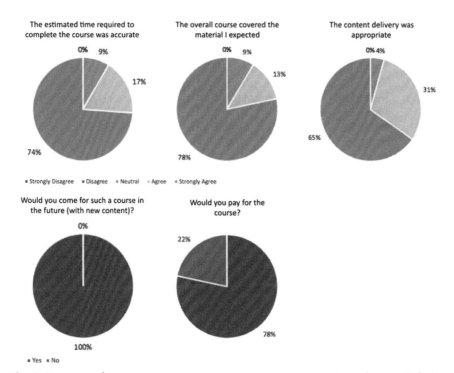

Fig. 3. Responses from an anonymous postcourse course survey to evaluate satisfaction level. N = 23 respondents. The term course refers to both online modules and hands-on sessions for C-OTS and BD-TTS techniques.

Our observations were made in a general hospital where physicians are salaried and reimbursement to the hospital based on the technology used was generally not an issue. Having such a setting is important to note because it adds to the many roadblocks that prevent new innovations from reaching patient care. Because reimbursement was not an issue in this particular observation, we were able to focus on the impact of learning.

Delivering the knowledge base and technical skills directly to the early majority allows them to self-learn the material at their own pace and to carefully evaluate the data related to the new technology, which they might need to do in order to decide if they will use C-OTS. We provide the early majority an extensive learning opportunity to reference themselves, because it is typically more difficult for them to reference early adopters when deciding to use new technology.[1,6] In fact, the early majority tends to feel alienated by the early adopters owing to the latter's (1) lack of respect for their colleagues' experiences; (2) greater interest in technology; (3) failure to recognize the importance of existing infrastructure; and (4) overall disruptiveness.

In gastroenterology, endoscopic skills acquisition typically occurs during fellowship, and practicing endoscopists have limited access to hands-on training and assessment. For our courses, we used a flipped learning framework in order to provide practicing physicians the opportunity to learn the application of OTS clips in the treatment of UGIB. We selected this pedagogy because it provides a basis for one of the most successful accelerated learning paradigms in the world: teenage driver's licensing. This training paradigm involves 6 systematic steps as outlined in **Fig. 2.**

Our curriculum for the C-OTS course integrates both the knowledge base and the technical skills required for practicing gastroenterologists and fellows to efficiently learn this new technology. Our use of a cloud-based LMS allowed us to simplify the process for disseminating information using different learning modalities, including instructional videos, high-quality images, and competency-based assessments. Our course design allowed us to ensure that the technical skills can only be learned after the cognitive knowledge is attained.

There are potential drawbacks of the learning system that we used. Creating their curriculum and learning content requires significant resources, time, and effort compared with the traditional method of passive teaching at the bedside. Many participants, who are used to passive learning via didactic lectures, initially expressed dissatisfaction at having to actively learn independently and being required to pass a self-assessment examination. However, most participants changed their views to have a more favorable opinion of the self-study modules after completing the experiential learning portion of the course.

In conclusion, our experience of using flipped learning to train this group of practicing gastroenterologists and fellows has encouraged the adoption of a relatively complex procedure, C-OTS, and of an established yet underutilized technique, endoscopic balloon dilation, within a short time period. The promising results suggest a robust flipped learning system may be useful to cross the chasm in the adoption of new technology in endoscopy.

ACKNOWLEDGMENTS

We express special thanks of gratitude to Jason Chang, MD, Mark De Lusong, MD, Thomas Gottwald, MD, PhD, Christopher Khor, MD, James Lau, MD, and Rungsun Rerknimitr, MD for their valuable contributions and support to this novel attempt at training a new technology.

Presented in part as an oral presentation at Digestive Disease Week (DDW) 2019.

REFERENCES

1. Moore G. Crossing the chasm. 3rd edition. New York: Harper Business Essentials; 2014.
2. Khateeb OM. The 4 stages to technology adoption inside the chasm. Medium 2017. Available at: https://medium.com/@omarmkhateeb/the-4-stages-to-adoption-inside-the-chasm-6c9c19e4375. Accessed August 28, 2019.
3. Baig MS, Mallu HS. Advances in medical education and practice: what millennial medical students say about flipped learning. Adv Med Educ Pract 2017;8:681–2.
4. Soetikno R, Kolb JM, Nguyen-Vu T, et al. Evolving endoscopy teaching in the era of the millennial trainee. Gastrointest Endosc 2019;89(5):1056–62.
5. ACGME program requirements for graduate medical education in gastroenterology (subspecialty of internal medicine). Accreditation Council for Graduate Medical Education (ACGME); 2019.
6. Linowes JS. A summary of "Crossing the Chasm" Parker Hill technology. Available at: https://ewthoff.home.xs4all.nl/Weppage%20documents/Summary%20Crossing%20the%20Chasm.pdf. Accessed August 28, 2019.

The Development of the Overstitch System and Its Potentials

Sergey V. Kantsevoy, MD, PhD

KEYWORDS

- Flexible endoscopy • Endoscopic suturing device
- Endoscopic mucosal resection (EMR) • Endoscopic submucosal dissection (ESD)
- Endoscopic bariatric procedures

KEY POINTS

- The predecessor of Overstitch system was the Eagle Claw device, which was only used in experiments on isolated pig stomachs and live porcine models.
- The first-generation Overstitch system was cleared by the FDA for clinical use in humans in 2008 and released for general use in the United States on October 18, 2010.
- The second-generation Overstitch system (compatible only with Olympus double-channel endoscopes) was launched in the United States on December 20, 2011, and is currently available on several continents (Asia, Australia, Europe, North and South America).
- The Overstitch Sx system, compatible with more than 20 single-channel flexible endoscopes with diameters ranging from 8.8 mm to 9.8 mm made by major endoscope manufacturers (eg, Olympus, Pentax, Fuji) was launched in November 2018 and is available for clinical use in humans in the United States and Europe.

INTRODUCTION

Multiple new devices and techniques were introduced into clinical practice at the beginning of the twenty-first century. But development of endoscopic suturing with the Overstitch device has changed the face of flexible endoscopy.

DEVELOPMENT OF OVERSTITCH ENDOSCOPIC SUTURING DEVICE AND INDICATIONS FOR ENDOSCOPIC SUTURING

The concept of a suturing device for flexible endoscopy was introduced by Apollo Group in partnership with Olympus Optical Ltd (Tokyo, Japan). The Apollo Group (**Fig. 1**) was a scientific collaboration of seven scientists from the United States and Hong Kong: Peter B. Cotton, MD and Robert H. Hawes, MD (Medical University of South Carolina, Charleston, SC), Anthony N. Kalloo, MD and Sergey V. Kantsevoy,

301 St Paul Place POB, Suite 718, Baltimore, MD 20202, USA
E-mail address: skan51@hotmail.com

Gastrointest Endoscopy Clin N Am 30 (2020) 107–114
https://doi.org/10.1016/j.giec.2019.08.004
1052-5157/20/© 2019 Elsevier Inc. All rights reserved.

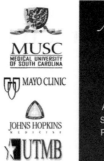
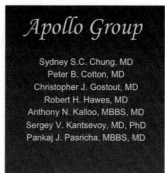

Fig. 1. The Apollo Group.

MD, PhD (Johns Hopkins University School of Medicine, Baltimore, MD), Christopher J. Gostout, MD (Mayo Clinic, Rochester, MN), Pankaj J. Pasricha, MD (University of Texas at Galveston, Galveston, TX), and Sydney S.C. Chung, MD (Chinese University of Hong Kong, Hong Kong, China).

The first meeting of Apollo Group was arranged and sponsored by Olympus Optical Ltd in South Carolina in 1999 (**Fig. 2**). During that meeting the group discussed limitations of existing flexible endoscopy and chose several prospective scientific projects: transgastric interventions inside the peritoneal cavity, widespread endoscopic mucosectomy for removal of Barrett esophagus, endoscopic correction of gastroesophageal reflux disease, endoscopic treatment of obesity, and development of endoscopic suturing device. All members of Apollo Group perceived endoscopic suturing device as a key necessary element for future advanced flexible endoscopic procedures.

Since the first meeting, the members of Apollo Group and dedicated engineers from Olympus Optical Ltd had regular meetings to discuss the progress in Apollo Group projects. Numerous patent applications were submitted including the patents for suturing systems for flexible endoscopy. Then the Olympus Corporation engineers made the first prototype of the endoscopic suturing device (**Fig. 3**A). The distal end of this device (**Fig. 3**B) had a plastic ring for mounting on the distal end of a single-channel upper endoscope. The distal end of the device resembled the claw of an eagle and was called Eagle Claw by professor Sydney S.C. Chung, MD. Eagle Claw allowed

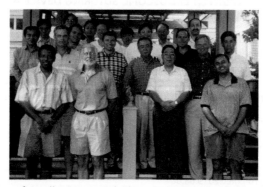

Fig. 2. First meeting of Apollo Group and Olympus Corporation in South Carolina, 1999.

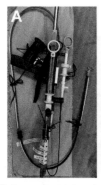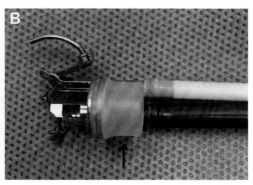

Fig. 3. (*A*) An endoscopic suturing device. (*B*) Distal end of the endoscopic suturing device: Single arrow demonstrates a plastic ring for mounting of the suturing device on the distal end of a single channel upper endoscope.

performance of a separate stitch with intracorporeal knot tying. The Eagle Claw was not designed to make continuous suturing line and required removal from the operating field after completion of each stitch. The new stitch was reloaded outside of the animal and then the endoscope with Eagle Claw was reinserted back into the operating field.

Eagle Claw was used in numerous bench top experiments on isolated pig stomachs and live porcine models and demonstrated technical feasibility of endoscopic suturing of bleeding ulcers, endoscopic restriction of the stomach (currently known as endoscopic sleeve gastroplasty), endoscopic correction of internal hernias, endoscopic creation of gastrojejunal anastomosis, and closure of the gastric entrance into the peritoneal cavity.[1–7]

Despite numerous modifications and improvements, Eagle Claw was not a user-friendly device. It required long and tedious assembly, and was never used in humans.

Apollo Group members in 2006 decided to form a company dedicated to development of an endoscopic suturing system. Dennis McWilliams was hired as President and CEO of a new company, Apollo Endosurgery. Mr McWilliams was able to raise necessary initial capital. He also hired upper management and engineers and created the company with headquarters and first production facility in Austin, Texas.

The first generation of Overstitch endoscopic suturing device was cleared by the Food and Drug Administration (FDA) in 2008 as a general-use device and released into clinical practice in the United States on October 18, 2010.

The first generation of Overstitch (**Fig. 4**A) was a bulky device requiring considerable assembly. The distal end (called end plate) of the first generation of Overstitch (**Fig. 4**B) had a straight tubular structure, which was inserted into the larger channel of the double-channel endoscope (Olympus GiF-2T160). To prevent detachment of the end plate from the endoscope, a metal wire was passed through the channel of the endoscope and attached to the special mounting hardware.

The device was able to create separate stitches and continuous suturing line with intracorporeal knot tying (cinching). After completion of the first suture, the suturing device could be reloaded with a new suture unlimited number of times without the need to remove the endoscope from the patient.

The first clinical use of the Overstitch in humans was published in 2012 by Kantsevoy and Thuluvath[8] for endoscopic correction of long-standing gastrocutaneous

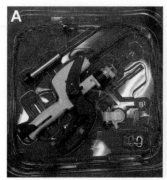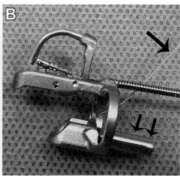

Fig. 4. First generation of the Overstitch endoscopic suturing system. (*A*) First generation of the Overstitch system in a package. (*B*) End plate of the first generation of the Overstitch system. *Single arrow* indicates a fixation wire attached to the end plate and *double arrows* demonstrate a straight tubular structure for insertion into the larger channel of double-channel Olympus upper endoscopes GiF-2T160 and GiF-2T180.

fistula post removal of percutaneous endoscopic gastrostomy feeding tube. Following this encouraging positive experience, similar result was successfully achieved in an immune-compromised patient.[9]

After initial case reports on closure of gastrocutaneous fistulas, a case series reporting the use of Overstitch for closure of recalcitrant marginal ulcers was published by Jirapinyo and coworkers.[10] Soon afterward a successful fixation of esophageal stents with Overstitch to prevent stent migration was independently reported by Kantsevoy and Bitner[11] and by Swanstrom and colleagues.[12] Endoscopic suturing to prevent migration of esophageal stents proved to be an effective technique and was subsequently independently validated by other researchers.[13]

The first generation of Overstitch was soon replaced by a second generation of the endoscopic suturing device (**Fig. 5**A), which was launched in the United States on December 20, 2011. This device consisted of a handle connected by accentuation cord to an end plate and a needle holder. The second generation of Overstitch was compatible only with Olympus GiF-2T160 and GiF-2T180 double-channel gastroscopes.

The second generation of Overstitch represented a major improvement of the suturing system: it was an easy to assemble, sleek, and user-friendly device. The end plate of the second generation of the Overstitch (**Fig. 5**B) had a tube with a built-in spring-loaded mechanism, which was inserted into the larger channel of a double-channel Olympus upper endoscope. The built-in spring-loaded mechanism prevented detachment of the end plate from the distal tip of the endoscope and eliminated the need for fixation wire present in the previous generation of the Overstitch system.

Introduction of the second generation of Overstitch into clinical practice resulted in a rapid expansion of clinical applications for its use. Currently widely used and well-established applications for endoscopic suturing include fixation of internal stents to prevent stent migration[11–13]; closure of large defects post endoscopic mucosal resection and endoscopic submucosal dissection (ESD)[14]; endoscopic closure of gastrointestinal tract perforations, fistulas, and anastomotic leaks[8,9,15–21]; closure of the tunnel entrance for peroral endoscopic myotomy and submucosal tunnel endoscopic resection[22–27]; and endoscopic bariatric procedures (repair of dilated

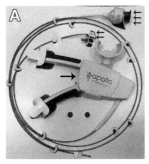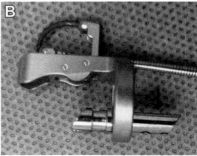

Fig. 5. Second generation of the Overstitch endoscopic suturing system. (*A*) Second generation of the Overstitch system in a package. *Single arrow* demonstrates a handle connected by accentuation cord to an end plate (*double arrows*). *Triple arrows* demonstrate a needle holder. (*B*) End plate of the second generation of the Overstitch system. *Single arrow* indicates a tube with a built-in spring-loaded mechanism for insertion into the larger channel of a double-channel Olympus upper endoscope.

gastrojejunal anastomosis post gastric bypass and primary endoscopic sleeve gastroplasty).[28–38]

Second generation of Overstitch is now available in several continents (Asia, Australia, Europe, North and South America). However, the second generation of Overstitch is only compatible with Olympus double-channel upper endoscopes. To construct a universal system compatible with multiple endoscope manufacturers (eg, Olympus, Pentax, Fuji), Apollo Endosurgery developed Overstich Sx system (**Fig. 6**A). The end plate of the Overstitch Sx (**Fig. 6**B) is fixed by two plastic strips to the distal end of a single-channel upper endoscope. Overstitch Sx system is compatible with more than 20 single-channel flexible endoscopes with diameters ranging from 8.8 mm to 9.8 mm made by major endoscope manufacturers (eg, Olympus, Pentax, Fuji). The end plate of the Overstitch Sx system has its own channels for tissue Helix device, needle and needle-holder leaving the working channel of the endoscope available for any additional accessories (eg, scissors, grasping forceps). The Overstitch Sx system was cleared by the FDA in November 2017 and launched in the United States in November 2018.

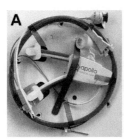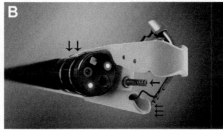

Fig. 6. Overstitch Sx for single-channel gastroscopes. (*A*) Overstitch Sx in a package. (*B*) End plate of the Overstitch Sx system. *Single arrow* demonstrates a dedicated channel for tissue Helix device. *Double arrows* indicate two plastic strips for fixation of the end plate to the distal end of a single-channel gastroscope. *Triple arrows* demonstrate a dedicated channel for needle and needle-holder. End plate of Overstitch Sx leaves the working channel of the endoscope available for any additional accessories (eg, scissors, grasping forceps). (*Courtesy of* Apollo Endosurgery, Inc, Austin, TX; with permission.)

In addition to well-established applications for endoscopic suturing, the list of new potential applications for use of Overstitch and Overstitch Sx systems is expanding and includes organ reconstruction post endoscopic and surgical interventions, treatment of gastroesophageal reflux disease, facilitation of ESD, and numerous other evolving indications.[39–41] Some of these indications are discussed in detail elsewhere in this issue.

SUMMARY

Development of Overstitch endoscopic suturing system changed the face of flexible endoscopy. Second generation of Overstitch is easy to assemble and to use, but it is only compatible with Olympus double-channel endoscopes (GiF-2T160 and GiF-2T180). The newest model, Overstitch Sx, is compatible with more than 20 single-channel flexible endoscopes with diameters ranging from 8.8 mm to 9.8 mm made by major endoscopes manufacturers (eg, Olympus, Pentax, Fuji).

Overstitch system is now approved for general clinical use on several continents (Asia, Australia, Europe, North and South America). The list of applications for endoscopic suturing is already long, but it continues to expand and include well-established procedures (fixation of internal stents, closure of anastomotic leaks, gastrointestinal tract fistulas and iatrogenic perforations, suturing closure of mucosal defects post endoscopic mucosal resection, ESD, submucosal tunnel endoscopic resection and peroral endoscopic myotomy, endoscopic hemostasis for bleeding ulcers, primary and secondary bariatric procedures) and new, evolving indications (eg, organ reconstruction post endoscopic and surgical interventions, treatment of gastroesophageal reflux disease, facilitation of ESD)

REFERENCES

1. Hu B, Chung SC, Sun LC, et al. Eagle Claw II: a novel endosuture device that uses a curved needle for major arterial bleeding: a bench study. Gastrointest Endosc 2005;62:266–70.
2. Hu B, Chung SC, Sun LC, et al. Developing an animal model of massive ulcer bleeding for assessing endoscopic hemostatic devices. Endoscopy 2005;37: 847–51.
3. Hu B, Chung SC, Sun LC, et al. Endoscopic suturing without extracorporeal knots: a laboratory study. Gastrointest Endosc 2005;62:230–3.
4. Hu B, Kalloo AN, Chung SS, et al. Peroral transgastric endoscopic primary repair of a ventral hernia in a porcine model. Endoscopy 2007;39:390–3.
5. Hu B, Chung SC, Sun LC, et al. Transoral obesity surgery: endoluminal gastroplasty with an endoscopic suture device. Endoscopy 2005;37:411–4.
6. Kantsevoy SV, Hu B, Jagannath SB, et al. Technical feasibility of endoscopic gastric reduction: a pilot study in a porcine model. Gastrointest Endosc 2007; 65:510–3.
7. Chiu PW, Hu B, Lau JY, et al. Endoscopic plication of massively bleeding peptic ulcer by using the Eagle Claw VII device: a feasibility study in a porcine model. Gastrointest Endosc 2006;63:681–5.
8. Kantsevoy SV, Thuluvath PJ. Successful closure of a chronic refractory gastrocutaneous fistula with a new endoscopic suturing device (with video). Gastrointest Endosc 2012;75:688–90.
9. Armengol-Miro JR, Dot J, Abu-Suboh Abadia M, et al. New endoscopic suturing device for closure of chronic gastrocutaneous fistula in an immunocompromised patient. Endoscopy 2012;43(Suppl 2 UCTN):E403–4.

10. Jirapinyo P, Watson RR, Thompson CC. Use of a novel endoscopic suturing device to treat recalcitrant marginal ulceration (with video). Gastrointest Endosc 2012;76:435–9.

11. Kantsevoy SV, Bitner M. Esophageal stent fixation with endoscopic suturing device (with video). Gastrointest Endosc 2012;76:1251–5.

12. Rieder E, Dunst CM, Martinec DV, et al. Endoscopic suture fixation of gastrointestinal stents: proof of biomechanical principles and early clinical experience. Endoscopy 2012;44:1121–6.

13. Sharaiha RZ, Kumta NA, DeFilippis EM, et al. A large multicenter experience with endoscopic suturing for management of gastrointestinal defects and stent anchorage in 122 patients: a retrospective review. J Clin Gastroenterol 2016; 50:388–92.

14. Kantsevoy SV, Bitner M, Mitrakov AA, et al. Endoscopic suturing closure of large mucosal defects after endoscopic submucosal dissection is technically feasible, fast, and eliminates the need for hospitalization (with videos). Gastrointest Endosc 2013;79:503–7.

15. Kantsevoy SV, Bitner M, Davis JM, et al. Endoscopic suturing closure of large iatrogenic colonic perforation. Gastrointest Endosc 2015;82:754–5.

16. Kantsevoy SV, Bitner M, Hajiyeva G, et al. Endoscopic management of colonic perforations: clips versus suturing closure (with videos). Gastrointest Endosc 2016;84(3):487–93.

17. Kumar N, Thompson CC. A novel method for endoscopic perforation management by using abdominal exploration and full-thickness sutured closure. Gastrointest Endosc 2014;80:156–61.

18. Bonin EA, Wong Kee Song LM, Gostout ZS, et al. Closure of a persistent esophagopleural fistula assisted by a novel endoscopic suturing system. Endoscopy 2012;44(Suppl 2 UCTN):E8–9.

19. Chon SH, Toex U, Plum PS, et al. Successful closure of a gastropulmonary fistula after esophagectomy using the Apollo Overstitch and endoscopic vacuum therapy. Endoscopy 2018;50:E149–50.

20. Henderson JB, Sorser SA, Atia AN, et al. Repair of esophageal perforations using a novel endoscopic suturing system. Gastrointest Endosc 2014;80:535–7.

21. Winder JS, Pauli EM. Comprehensive management of full-thickness luminal defects: the next frontier of gastrointestinal endoscopy. World J Gastrointest Endosc 2015;7:758–68.

22. Stavropoulos SN, Modayil R, Friedel D, et al. Endoscopic full-thickness resection for GI stromal tumors. Gastrointest Endosc 2014;80:334–5.

23. Stavropoulos SN, Modayil R, Friedel D. Current applications of endoscopic suturing. World J Gastrointest Endosc 2015;7:777–89.

24. Kantsevoy SV. Endoscopic suturing for closure of transmural defects. Tech Gastrointest Endosc 2015;17:136–40.

25. Kantsevoy SV, Armengol-Miro JR. Endoscopic suturing, an essential enabling technology for new NOTES interventions. Gastrointest Endosc Clin N Am 2016; 26:375–84.

26. Armengol-Miro JR, Dot Bach J, Suboh Abadia MA, et al. Natural orifice translimenal endoscopic surgery (NOTES) for G.I. tract neoplasia. In: Testoni PA, Arcidiacono PG, Mariani A, editors. Endoscopic management of gastrointestinal cancer and precancerous conditions. Turin (Italy): Edizoni Minerva Medica; 2015. p. 277–83.

27. Pescarus R, Shlomovitz E, Sharata AM, et al. Endoscopic suturing versus endoscopic clip closure of the mucosotomy during a per-oral endoscopic myotomy (POEM): a case-control study. Surg Endosc 2016;30:2132–5.

28. Kantsevoy SV. Endoscopic suturing devices. In: Testoni PA, Arcidiacono PG, Mariani A, editors. Endoscopic management of gastrointestinal cancer and precancerous conditions. Turin (Italy): Edizoni Minerva Medica; 2015. p. 249–55.

29. Conway NE, Swanstrom LL. Endoluminal flexible endoscopic suturing for minimally invasive therapies. Gastrointest Endosc 2014;81:262–9.e19.

30. Sartoretto A, Sui Z, Hill C, et al. Endoscopic sleeve gastroplasty (ESG) is a reproducible and effective endoscopic bariatric therapy suitable for widespread clinical adoption: a large, international multicenter study. Obes Surg 2018;28: 1812–21.

31. Khan Z, Khan MA, Hajifathalian K, et al. Efficacy of endoscopic interventions for the management of obesity: a meta-analysis to compare endoscopic sleeve gastroplasty, AspireAssist, and primary obesity surgery endolumenal. Obes Surg 2019;29:2287–98.

32. Lopez-Nava G, Galvao MP, da Bautista-Castano I, et al. Endoscopic sleeve gastroplasty for the treatment of obesity. Endoscopy 2015;47:449–52.

33. Lopez-Nava G, Galvao MP, Bautista-Castano I, et al. Endoscopic sleeve gastroplasty for obesity treatment: two years of experience. Arq Bras Cir Dig 2017;30: 18–20.

34. Lopez-Nava G, Sharaiha RZ, Vargas EJ, et al. Endoscopic sleeve gastroplasty for obesity: a multicenter study of 248 patients with 24 months follow-up. Obes Surg 2017;27:2649–55.

35. Abu Dayyeh BK, Neto MG, Lopez-Nava G, et al. Endoscopic sleeve gastroplasty is safe and effective: pitfalls of a flawed systematic review. Surg Obes Relat Dis 2019. [Epub ahead of print].

36. Schulman AR, Huseini M, Thompson CC. Endoscopic sleeve gastroplasty of the remnant stomach in Roux-en-Y gastric bypass: a novel approach to a gastrogastric fistula with weight regain. Endoscopy 2018;50:E132–3.

37. Barrichello S Jr, Hourneaux de Moura DT, Hourneaux de Moura EG, et al. Endoscopic sleeve gastroplasty in the management of overweight and obesity: an international multicenter study. Gastrointest Endosc 2019. [Epub ahead of print].

38. de Moura DTH, de Moura EGH, Thompson CC. Endoscopic sleeve gastroplasty: from whence we came and where we are going. World J Gastrointest Endosc 2019;11:322–8.

39. Rieder E, Makris KI, Martinec DV, et al. The suture-pulley method for endolumenal triangulation in endoscopic submucosal dissection. Endoscopy 2011;43(Suppl 2 UCTN):E319–20.

40. Aihara H, Kumar N, Ryou M, et al. Facilitating endoscopic submucosal dissection: the suture-pulley method significantly improves procedure time and minimizes technical difficulty compared with conventional technique: an ex vivo study (with video). Gastrointest Endosc 2014;80:495–502.

41. Kantsevoy SV, Wagner A, Mitrakov AA, et al. Rectal reconstruction after endoscopic submucosal dissection for removal of a giant rectal lesion. VideoGIE 2019;4:179–81.

The Use of the Overstitch for Bariatric Weight Loss

Rabindra R. Watson, MD*

KEYWORDS

- Endoscopic suturing • Endoscopic sleeve gastroplasty • Transoral outlet reduction

KEY POINTS

- The advent and widespread availability of a commercially available full-thickness suturing device has led to the creation of novel endoscopic gastric plication procedures for the management of obesity.
- A growing body of literature supports endoscopic sleeve gastroplasty as an effective, safe, and reproducible minimally invasive treatment for obesity and metabolic disease.
- Weight regain with return of metabolic diseases after bariatric surgery is common and can be managed with endoscopic suturing.
- Endoscopic suturing techniques such as transoral outlet reduction can repair postbariatric surgical anatomic aberrations such as gastrojejunal anastomosis aperture dilation that contribute to weight gain.
- Endoscopic sutured bariatric techniques should only be performed in the context of a comprehensive, multidisciplinary weight management program.

 Video content accompanies this article at http://www.giendo.theclinics.com.

INTRODUCTION

Obesity is a public health pandemic and a leading contributor to morbidity and mortality in the United States and worldwide.[1,2] A steady increase in the prevalence of obesity has been observed over the past 20 years, resulting in a significant burden on health care resources and costs.[3] Diet and lifestyle programs have demonstrated limited efficacy with respect to clinically meaningful weight loss and weight recidivism rates remain high.[4,5] Several pharmacotherapies have been approved by the US Food and Drug Administration for long-term weight management, and modest weight loss has been demonstrated in several clinical trials. However long-term data are limited, and side effects, cost, and adherence remain a concern.[6] Bariatric surgeries such

Disclosure Statement: Dr R.R. Watson receives consulting fees from Apollo Endosurgery, Boston Scientific, and Neptune Medical.
Interventional Endoscopy Services, California Pacific Medical Center, University of California, San Francisco, San Francisco, CA, USA
* 1101 Van Ness Avenue, Room 3158, San Francisco, CA 94109.
E-mail address: watsorr@sutterhealth.org

as the laparoscopic sleeve gastrectomy (LSG) and Roux-en-Y gastric bypass (RYGB) are effective, although they have achieved limited penetration owing in part to invasiveness, cost, and availability.[7,8]

Endoscopic bariatric therapies have emerged as viable minimally invasive treatment options to fill the therapeutic gap between conservative and surgical approaches. A variety of techniques have been described, many of which emulate surgical approaches such as gastric restriction or intestinal bypass. The evolution of endoscopic suturing technology has resulted in the ability to reliably place full-thickness sutures throughout the gastrointestinal tract, opening the door to novel endoscopic gastric restrictive procedures. Such endoscopic procedures include primary treatments for obesity such as the endoscopic sleeve gastroplasty (ESG), as well as revisional procedures including transoral outlet reduction (TORe) and endoscopic sleeve revision for the treatment of weight regain following RYGB and LSG, respectively.

PRIMARY WEIGHT LOSS THERAPY
Suction-Based Suturing

The primary endoscopic treatment of obesity using suturing techniques was first described in 2006 using a suction-based suturing device (Bard EndoCinch, Davol, Murray Hill, NJ). The technique involved the placement of longitudinal endoscopic plications along the anterior and posterior surfaces of the gastric body using a single suture to create an endoscopic vertical gastroplasty, analogous to a vertical banded gastroplasty.[9] Although the initial results seemed promising, the technique was limited by superficial tissue plication and the need to remove the device from the patient to reload sutures.

The device was subsequently modified to eliminate the need for ex vivo suture reloading and to obtain deeper tissue plications (RESTORe Suturing System, Bard). Additionally, the technique was modified to use a series of running stitches that incorporate the greater curvature analogous to surgical gastric imbrication. This approach may be regarded as the forerunner of ESG. In an 18-patient feasibility study, gastric plications were completed successfully in all patients.[10] A 12-month follow-up study of the same cohort including 14 patients demonstrated a mean percent excess weight loss (%EWL) of 27.7% $\pm$ 21.9% as well as significant decreases in waist circumference and systolic blood pressure. However, partial or complete release of the plications were observed in 13 of 14 patients during endoscopy performed at 1 year.[11]

Full-Thickness Suturing

The Overstitch device (Apollo Endosurgery, Austin, TX) has improved on suction-based tissue plication by using a curved needle driver as well as a mechanical tissue retractor (Helix) to ensure reliable, full-thickness tissue acquisition and plication. The device may be used to create a variety of suture patterns including interrupted or running stitches, as well as more complex configurations such as vest-over-pants, figure-of-8, and purse-string stitches. Furthermore, suture reloading does not necessitate device removal from the patient. The Overstitch is US Food and Drug Administration cleared for tissue apposition in the gastrointestinal tract and has been used for a variety of indications, such as defect closure, stent fixation, and bariatric indications.[12] The device was originally only compatible with a 2 accessory channel endoscope, however a single channel iteration has recently become available (Overstitch SX, Apollo Endosurgery). Nonabsorbable 2-0 polypropylene and absorbable 2-0 polydioxanone suture is available.

Endoscopic Sleeve Gastroplasty

The technique for ESG was developed as part of a 3 phase international multicenter trial initiated in 2012.[13] The first phase consisted of assessment of safety and technical feasibility of procedure techniques including various stitch patterns in an initial cohort consisting of 5 patients. In this context, an initial US single-center study was also published including 4 patients. Two layers of interrupted plications were created along the gastric body, and the fundus was also closed with a 2-layer sutured technique. The mean procedure length was 212.5 minutes, and a mean of 25.5 sutures were used.[14] The technique was iteratively refined and the preferred technique then evaluated in a 2 center 22 patient cohort in phase II. Procedural modifications included the use of a triangular running stitch pattern and restriction of the plications to the gastric corpus with preservation of the fundic reservoir. The third phase evaluated the technical feasibility of the technique as well as perioperative care and weight loss outcomes in an international cohort of 77 patients as part of an international prospective registry. Patients had a mean age of 41.3 $\pm$ 1.1 years and the mean body mass index (BMI) was 36.1 $\pm$ 0.6 kg/m^2. The mean percent total body weight loss (%TBWL) was 16.0 $\pm$ 0.8% at 6 months and 17.4 $\pm$ 1.2% at 12 months of follow-up (n = 44). Although epigastric pain and nausea were frequently reported in the first week after the procedure, no serious adverse events were reported.

Patient selection

In clinical studies, ESG has been offered to patients with a BMI of 30 to 40 kg/m^2 who have failed attempts at diet and lifestyle modification. Exclusion criteria typically include patients with a coagulation disorder, history of gastric surgery, large hiatus hernia (>3 cm), foregut inflammatory bowel disease, peptic ulcer disease, eating disorders, and active psychiatric disease. Importantly, patients must also demonstrate a commitment to a longitudinal weight loss management program.

Procedural technique

- Patients are typically placed under general endotracheal intubation.
- The use of an esophageal overtube may aid in initial intubation of the esophagus with the Overstitch device, and facilitate scope reinsertion if necessary during the procedure.
- Administration of a prophylactic broad-spectrum antibiotic, such as a third-generation cephalosporin is recommended.
- Intraoperative prophylactic antiemetics such as ondansetron, prochlorperazine, metoclopramide, and dexamethasone, are often administered. Preprocedure placement of a scopolamine patch and administration of aprepitant may also be considered.
- Intraoperative venous thromboembolic prophylaxis should be considered owing to the bariatric patient population and longer procedure times, particularly during the initial learning phase.
- Carbon dioxide insufflation is mandatory owing to the full-thickness nature of suture placement and resultant pneumoperitoneum.
- After diagnostic endoscopy, the anterior and posterior margins for suture placement along the anterior and posterior walls may be marked using argon plasma coagulation at standard settings.
- A basic consensus procedural technique is most widely performed and taught through industry and society-sponsored courses. However, minor site-specific variations in technique exist.

○ Running stitches are placed in a distal to proximal fashion from the proximal antrum/incisura to the proximal corpus. The fundus is typically not incorporated owing to risks of perigastric peritoneal organ injury and the technical complexity of suturing in the semiflexed or fully retroflexed position.

○ The use of the tissue helix is recommended for the acquisition of all tissue plications to ensure consistent full-thickness stitches and avoidance of peritoneal organ injury.

○ A triangular stitch pattern is used, spanning from the anterior wall to the greater curvature to the posterior wall. A series of 6 stitch placements consisting of 2 triangles in series is placed and the suture is then cinched. This results in exclusion of the greater curvature while also shortening the length of the stomach, resulting in a tubular sleeve along the length of the lesser curvature (**Fig. 1**).

○ Care should be taken to avoid the formation of gaps or longitudinal furrows along the greater curvature. Varying the sites of tissue plications along the greater curvature during the creation of adjacent triangles may mitigate this issue.

○ A second medial line of either interrupted or running stitches may be placed to further reduce the gastric volume and/or reinforce the initial running stitches.

○ Frequent reassessment of the modified anatomy during sleeve creation is recommended to avoid stenosis or angulation within the sleeve lumen.

○ A varying number of sutures is used, typically between 6 and 9 per case.

Postprocedure care

• Patients are observed in the postprocedure unit and given intravenous antiemetics and analgesia as needed.

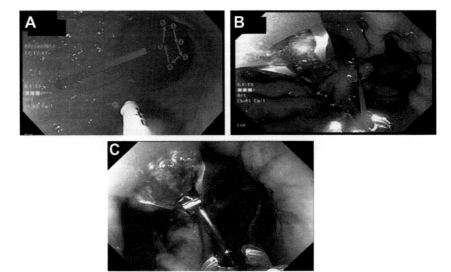

Fig. 1. ESG procedure. (*A*) Marking of anterior and posterior border of suture line with Argon plasma coagulation, and diagram of planned stitch sites (*blue arrow* and *blue numbering*). (*B*) Creation of sleeve using the Overstitch device. (*C*) Final construct as viewed from the gastroesophageal junction with fundic cap visible to the left and sleeve lumen along the lesser curvature on the right. (*Courtesy of* Apollo Endosurgery, Austin, TX.)

- Generous administration of intravenous fluids should also be considered as patients are kept nil per os from the night before to 1 day after the procedure.
- Patients are provided with prescriptions for oral antiemetics, analgesics, antispasmodics, and a proton pump inhibitor upon discharge. Ideally, patients will have obtained these prescriptions prior the procedure to ensure adherence.
- Patients are discharged home the day of procedure. Rarely, patients may be admitted for observation in the setting of persistent abdominal pain or nausea.
- A staged diet is prescribed with progression from clear liquids, full liquids, soft solid foods, to a solid diet over the course of 6 to 8 weeks.
- Adherence to a postprocedure comprehensive weight loss program is critical to weight loss success. The number of follow-up visits to the multidisciplinary team (eg, nutrition, psychology) has been shown to be a predictor of weight loss outcomes.[15]

Mechanism

Despite the similarity in nomenclature between ESG and LSG, there are several important mechanistic differences between the 2 procedures. First, LSG permanently alters the gastric anatomy via resection of the gastric corpus and fundus, whereas the ESG results in a form of gastric imbrication. Therefore, gastrectomy results in removal of ghrelin producing cells and theoretically results in more durable weight loss. However, ESG is potentially reversible as well as repeatable, and may also result in short-term reductions in fasting and postprandial serum ghrelin levels.[16] The less invasive nature of ESG also results in lower morbidity.[17]

The mechanistic difference between these procedures is further highlighted by their contrasting effects on gastric motility. LSG has been shown to accelerate gastric emptying, which may in turn may alter secretion of gut hormones.[18] In contrast, in a study of 25 patients undergoing ESG, 4 of whom were subjected to physiologic analyses including gastric scintigraphy, an increase in time for 50% emptying of solid by 90 minutes ($P = .03$) was observed. Notably, there was no significant reduction in gastric emptying of liquids ($P = .5$).[16] Interestingly, 32.25% of the meal was retained in the small gastric fundus cap after ESG compared with 5.25% before the procedure.

Clinical data

- An initial US pilot series including 10 patients with a mean BMI of 45.2 kg/m^2 reported a mean EWL of 30% and mean absolute weight loss of 33 kg at 6 months.[19]
- A single-center study including 25 patients with a mean BMI of 38.5 $\pm$ 4.6 kg/m^2 reported a %TWL of 18.7 $\pm$ 10.7% at 12 months. In 1 patient, the procedure was revised for inadequate weight loss. In linear regression analysis adjusted by initial BMI, the frequency of nutritional ($\beta = 0.563$; $P = .014$) and psychological contacts ($\beta = 0.727$; $P = .025$) were associated with %TBWL.[15]
- An international, 3 - center study included 248 patients (mean age, 44.5 $\pm$ 10 years; 73% female). At 6 and 24 months, the %TBWL was 15.2% (95% confidence interval [CI], 14.2–16.3) and 18.6 (95% CI, 15.7–21.5), respectively. Weight loss was comparable between centers suggesting reproducibility of ESG between operators.[20]
- A second international 3 center study including 112 patients with a baseline BMI of 37.9 $\pm$ 6.7 kg/m^2 demonstrated a %TBWL of 14.9 $\pm$ 6.1% at 6 months. Weight loss was comparable between centers. Multivariate analysis suggested that male

sex, greater baseline body weight, and lack of prior endoscopic bariatric therapy were predictors of greater weight loss.[21]

- ESG has also been shown to improve metabolic complications of obesity. A single-center study of 91 consecutive patients with a mean BMI of 40.7 ± 7.0 kg/m² reported weight loss outcomes of 14.4% at 6 months (80% follow-up rate), 17.6% at 12 months (76% follow-up rate), and 20.9% at 24 months (66% follow-up rate). Moreover, at 12 months after ESG, patients experienced significant decreases in hemoglobin A1c (P = .01), systolic blood pressure (P = .02), waist circumference (P<.001), alanine aminotransferase (P<.001), and serum triglycerides (P = .02).[22] No significant reduction in low-density lipoprotein cholesterol was noted. A single perigastric leak occurred that was managed nonoperatively.
- The largest published series to date included 1000 patients from a single center with a baseline BMI of 33.3 ± 4.5 kg/m².[23] The mean %TWL (percent follow-up rate) at 6, 12, and, 18 months was 13.7 ± 6.8% (87.2%), 15.0 ± 7.7% (93.1%), and 14.8 ± 8.5 (85.7%), respectively. Short-term improvement in comorbidities was observed with 13 of 17 cases of diabetes (76%), 28/28 cases of hypertension (100%), and 18/32 cases of dyslipidemia (56%) achieving remission by the third month. Of note, 13 patients underwent either redo ESG (n = 5, mean nadir %TWL of 8.4 ± 2.8% at a mean of 166.4 days), or conversion to LSG (n = 8) for inadequate weight loss defined as a %TWL of less than 5% after 6 months. Significant adverse events requiring readmission occurred in 2.4% of patients:
  ○ Eight patients with significant abdominal pain, 3 of whom had ESG reversal;
  ○ Seven patients with bleeding, 2 of whom required transfusion;
  ○ Four patients with a perigastric collection with pleural effusion, 3 of whom underwent percutaneous drainage;
  ○ Five patients with postprocedure fever with no further sequelae.
- The durability of ESG has been evaluated in a single-center longitudinal study including 154 patients. Of the original cohort, 28 completed the 24-month assessment at which point the mean BMI changed from 38.3 to 30.8 kg/m² and %TBWL was 19.5%.[24]
- ESG has been compared with both laparoscopic adjustable gastric banding (LAGB) and LSG. A study conducted at a tertiary referral center included 278 obese (BMI >30) patients who underwent ESG (n = 91), LSG (n = 120), or LAGB (n = 67).[17] LSG demonstrated significantly greater %TBWL compared with LAGB and ESG (29.28% vs 13.30% vs 17.57%, respectively; P<.001). However, ESG demonstrated significantly lower morbidity compared with LSG and LAGB (P = .01), as well as significantly shorter length of hospital compared with LSG or LAGB (0.34 ± 0.73 days vs 3.09 ± 1.47 days vs 1.66 ± 3.07 days, respectively; P<.01).
- A second single-center matched cohort analysis compared ESG with LSG. A total of 54 ESG patients were matched with 83 LSG patients by age, sex, and BMI.[25] LSG resulted in significantly greater weight loss (23.6% ± 7.6% vs 17.1% ± 6.5%; P<.01), whereas ESG patients had significantly lower rates of adverse events (5.2% vs 16.9%; P<.05). Notably, new-onset gastroesophageal reflux disease was also significantly lower in the ESG group compared with the LSG group (1.9% vs 14.5%; P<.05). Given the known association of LSG with new-onset symptomatic gastroesophageal reflux disease and Barrett's esophagus, this study provides intriguing evidence for ESG as an alternative weight loss intervention in those patients at risk for such complications.

- The suture pattern of ESG has been recently modified and evaluated in a single center study including 148 patients with a mean BMI was 35.11 $\pm$ 5.5 kg/m^2.[26] A longitudinal Z stitch pattern was placed along the gastric body in 4 parallel rows. This stich pattern was chosen to distribute the suture tension more evenly and minimize suture breakage over time. A subgroup of 72 patients were followed for 18 months and demonstrated %TWL of a17.53% $\pm$ 7.57% at 12 months and 18.5% $\pm$ 9% at 18 months, demonstrating durability of this approach. Mild intraprocedural bleeding was noted in 1 case, which resolved with sclerotherapy.

Education and credentialing

Performing the ESG procedure requires knowledge of therapeutic endoscopic techniques including endoscopic hemostasis, familiarity with scope maneuvering/torqueing, Overstitch device set up and operation, as well as suture management. Currently, a specific recognized certification in ESG does not exist. Rather, training in ESG as part of a comprehensive endoscopic suturing program may be obtained through society or industry-sponsored courses. Likewise, credentialing in the ESG procedure is institution specific. Proctoring in initial cases is recommended, although it may not be mandatory, particularly for those operators with prior demonstrable facility with the Overstitch device.

Few data currently exist regarding the learning curve for ESG. The primary confounding factor in studying this issue is the operator's prior experience with the Overstitch device. Many new operators performing ESG have little to no prior experience with endoscopic suturing and therefore must gain general facility with the device concomitantly with learning the specific ESG procedure. In contrast, most high-volume centers have operators with extensive experience with the device for a variety of indications, and therefore the learning curve in this setting is primarily focused on procedural efficiency rather than safety or competence.

A study of the ESG learning curve included a single operator at an academic referral center with prior experience in endoscopic suturing who attended a 1-day ESG training course. Outcomes were measured in 21 consecutive ESG patients. The primary outcome measures were length of procedure and number of sutures used. The length of procedure decreased significantly across all procedures, with a learning plateau at 101.5 minutes and a learning rate of 7 cases ($P = .04$). The number of sutures used also decreased significantly over consecutive procedures, with a plateau at 8 sutures and a learning rate of 9 cases ($P<.001$). The average time per plication also decreased significantly with consecutive procedures, reaching a plateau at 9 procedures ($P<.001$).[27]

A second single-center study evaluated the learning curve in an operator with previous facility with the Overstitch device in 128 ESG patients performed at a tertiary referral center.[28] Efficiency (refining performance to decrease procedure time) and mastery (absence of outliers) were evaluated by using a penalized basis-spline regression and cumulative sum analysis. Efficiency was attained after 38 ESGs, with mastery achieved after 55 procedures. Notably, the endoscopist achieving efficiency was not correlated with successful weight loss at 12 months in multivariate analysis.

Beyond technical procedural considerations, the creation and implementation of a multidisciplinary weight management program is critical to optimal patient outcomes. Key components include a bariatric nutritionist, psychologist, and medical bariatrician or endocrinologist. A nurse navigator may also assist in patient outreach and coordination. Institutional support for such a program in coordination with existing bariatric surgery resources is ideal, although not mandatory. Gastroenterologists without such resources may partner with existing weight loss practices to provide comprehensive services. Operators should also be familiar with weight management principles and the perioperative care of the bariatric patient with appropriate unit infrastructure in place.

ENDOSCOPIC REVISION OF BARIATRIC SURGERY

Weight regain after bariatric surgery is an increasingly common referral indication for revision operations. Up to 30% of patients experience significant weight regain with return of comorbid diseases, and 20% fail to achieve at least 50% EWL at 1 year postoperatively.[29–31] Weight regain is further complicated by a negative impact on patient quality of life and increased health care-related costs.[32] The cause is likely multifactorial and includes maladaptive eating behaviors, lack of exercise, and postoperative neurohormonal changes over time, as well as postoperative anatomic changes. As the postbariatric surgery population grows over time, safe and cost-effective interventions to combat postoperative weight gain are increasingly needed.

Revision operations such as conversions to alternative bariatric operations, stomal revision, and/or distalization procedures have demonstrated efficacy in the treatment of weight gain or primary weight loss failure.[30,31,33,34] However, they are associated with a significant increase in perioperative morbidity and mortality compared with the index operation, likely owing to the presence of postoperative adhesions and surgically altered anatomy in a bariatric patient population.[35–38] There has, therefore, been considerable interest in alternative, nonoperative interventions targeting postoperative structural abnormalities that may contribute to weight regain. The primary focus of such investigations has been on revision of bypass operations.

Several cohort studies have demonstrated a significant correlation between both postoperative pouch size and gastrojejunal anastomosis (GJA) diameter and weight loss outcomes after RYGB. A single-center study evaluated 380 RYGB patients undergoing upper endoscopy at a mean postoperative interval of 5.9 ± 4.0 years. Among patients with a complaint of weight regain, the pouch and stoma size were normal in size (<6 cm long or <5 cm wide, <2 cm in diameter, respectively) in only 28.8% compared with 63.4% of those without weight regain ($P<.001$). In multivariate analysis, stoma diameter was independently associated with weight regain.[39] A subsequent single center study including 165 patients, 64% of whom experienced significant weight regain (≥20% of maximum weight lost after the RYGB), demonstrated that stomal diameter was the greatest predictor of weight regain on multivariable logistic regression analysis. Furthermore, a linear relationship between stomal aperture size and weight regain was demonstrated, suggesting a diameter of 15 mm or greater as clinically relevant dilation.[40]

Transoral Outlet Reduction

A variety of approaches have been used in the endoscopic treatment of weight regain after RYGB with targeting of GJA dilation. These methods include sclerotherapy or argon plasma coagulation to induce cicatrization of the GJA, gastric plication devices, and endoscopic suturing.[41] The feasibility and safety of TORe was initially reported in 2006 using a suction-based suturing system.[42] A subsequent randomized, sham-controlled multicenter trial using the same device demonstrated significantly greater weight loss in the TORe group (3.5%; 95% CI, 1.8%-5.3% vs 0.4%; 95% CI, 2.3% weight gain to 3.0% weight loss; $P = .021$), as well as improvements in metabolic parameters, thus establishing the feasibility and efficacy of TORe.[43]

The introduction of the Overstitch system has allowed for placement of full-thickness suture placement, with resultant superior durability. A single-center matched cohort study compared the suction-based device to the Overstitch in 118 TORe patients. Greater weight loss was observed in the full-thickness cohort at both the 6-month interval (10.6 ± 1.8 kg vs 4.4 ± 0.8 kg; $P<.01$), and the 12-month interval (8.6 ± 2.5 kg vs 2.9 ± 1.0 kg; $P<.01$).

It should be noted that, although reports also exist describing endoscopic suturing for gastric sleeve volume reduction after LSG, there is a dearth of literature regarding this approach and further study is warranted.[44]

Patient Selection

Owing to the chronic, relapsing nature of obesity and metabolic disease combined with the multifactorial etiology of weight regain, endoscopic revision should be offered only as part of a comprehensive weight management strategy. Key components of the preprocedure evaluation include the following.

- Nutritional consultation with review of eating behaviors and counseling as appropriate.
- Psychological evaluation and implementation of lifestyle interventions as appropriate.
- Evaluation for medical conditions that may contribute to weight gain such as:
  o Thyroid or other endocrine disease
  o Medications such as certain psychotropic medications, initiation of insulin, or beta blockers
- Evaluation and counseling for the initiation of weight loss medications in conjunction with endoscopic revision.
- Review of prior operative and endoscopic reports to determine the postoperative anatomy. Consideration of a preprocedure upper gastrointestinal study to determine anatomy and presence of a gastrogastric fistula may be considered.

Patients with return of obesity after RYGB or failure of the operation, often defined as failure to achieve 50% EWL at 1 year, should be considered for endoscopic revision. In addition, those patients who experience recrudescence of obesity-related metabolic disease such as diabetes, hypertension, dyslipidemia, obstructive sleep apnea, or fatty liver disease should also be considered as potential candidates, regardless of absolute weight.

Revision Technique

- The perioperative care of endoscopic revision patients is similar to that for ESG patients as outlined elsewhere in this article.
- The use of an esophageal overtube may aid in initial intubation of the esophagus with the Overstitch device, and facilitate scope reinsertion if necessary during the procedure.
- Intraoperative prophylactic antiemetics such as ondansetron, prochlorperazine, metoclopramide, and/or dexamethasone, are often administered. Preprocedure placement of a scopolamine patch and administration of aprepitant may also be considered.
- Carbon dioxide insufflation is mandatory owing to the full-thickness nature of suture placement and the possibility of pneumoperitoneum.
- After diagnostic endoscopy, the mucosa at the gastric aspect of the stoma is ablated using argon plasma coagulation (forced coagulation, 0.8–1.2 L/min, 30–50 W) to promote tissue apposition.

- Generally, a purse-string suture is placed around the GJA to reduce the aperture, although interrupted stitches may be placed. A purse-string is preferred owing superior force distribution over the sutures, which may mitigate suture breakage, lead to smaller aperture sizes, and result in better weight loss outcomes.[45]
- Stitches are placed with the suturing device placed across the GJA with the needle driven from the jejunal to the gastric aspect (**Fig. 2**, Video 1). The purse-string is achieved by torqueing the endoscope around the GJA, which may be technically challenging. Anywhere from 6 to 12 stitches are placed depending on the size of the outlet. Care should be taken to avoid suture crossing.
- Although an aperture diameter of less than 10 mm is desirable, excessive stomal reduction must be avoided to prevent symptomatic stenosis and suture loss. An 8-mm esophageal balloon dilator may be placed through the GJA during the cinching step to ensure uniform stomal sizing.
- A second layer of stitches may be placed in the distal pouch for reinforcement of the initial purse-string and for pouch reduction if needed.

Revision Data

- An initial case series including 25 patients demonstrated the safety and feasibility of the use of the Overstitch for TORe. Aperture reduction from 26.4 to 6.0 mm was achieved, with weight loss of 11.7 kg (69.5% of the regained weight was lost) at 6 months with no significant adverse events.[46]
- A meta-analysis including 330 patients demonstrated a pooled weight loss of 8.4 kg (95% CI, 6.5–10.3) at 18 to 24 months. Common adverse events included nausea (18%), abdominal pain (14%), and GJA stenosis requiring balloon dilation (5%).[47]

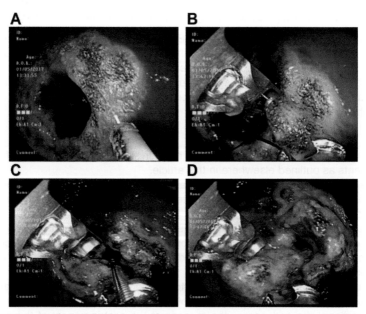

Fig. 2. TORe procedure. (*A*) Ablation of gastric mucosa at the GJA. (*B*) purse-string stitch placed using the Overstitch device. (*C*) Cinching of purse-string suture. (*D*) Final GJA construct after TORe. (*Courtesy of* Apollo Endosurgery, Austin, TX.)

- A single-center retrospective study compared outcomes between the interrupted (n = 54) or purse-string (n = 187) techniques.[48] At 12 months, the purse-string group achieved significantly greater weight loss: %TBWL (8.6 vs 6.4; P = .02), %EWL (19.8 vs 11.7; P<.001), total weight loss (9.5 vs 7.8; P = .04). Multivariable regression analysis demonstrated that technique was an independent predictor of %TBWL at 12 months, supporting the adoption of the purse-string technique as the preferred technique for TORe.
- A 3-center series including 130 consecutive patients subjected to TORe (mean age, 47 years; mean BMI, 36.8) demonstrated mean weight lost at 6, 12, and 18 months of 9.31 ± 6.70 kg (n = 84), 7.75 ± 8.40 kg (n = 70), 8.0 ± 8.8 kg (n = 46) (P<.01 for all 3 time points), respectively.[47]
- The durability of TORe has been demonstrated in a single center study of 150 patients with a mean preprocedure BMI of 40.2 ± 0.8 kg/m^2 presenting 8.6 ± 0.3 years after RYGB. Patients had regained of 49.9 ± 3.6% of their maximum lost weight. Weight loss was 10.5 ± 1.2 kg (24.9 ± 2.6% EWL) at 1 year, 9.0 ± 1.7 kg (20.0% ± 6.4% EWL) at 2 years, and 9.5 ± 2.1 kg (19.2% ± 4.6% EWL) at 3 years.[49] The number needed to treat to maintain weight loss of 5 kg or more from TORe was 1.2 at 6 months, 1.5 at 1 year, 1.9 at 2 years, and 2.0 at 3 years. Adverse events requiring emergency evaluation or admission included abdominal pain (4%), bleeding (hematemesis or melena) 3.3%, and nausea 2%.
- A subsequent 5-year follow-up study from the same institution included 50 patients (mean BMI 41.6 ± 10.7 kg/m^2), 37 of whom underwent TORe with an interrupted suture pattern; the remainder received a purse-string pattern.[50] At 5 years (76% follow-up rate), weight loss was 10.0 ± 15.1 kg (P = .0003) or 6.1 ± 9 % TBWL, with a BMI of 29.0 ± 16.9 kg/m^2 (P<.0001). The number needed to treat to stop weight regain at 1, 3, and 5 years was 1.1, 1.3, and 1.4, respectively. On a multivariate linear regression, the amount of weight regain was found to be predictive of %TBWL at 5 years after controlling for GJA size and number of stitches. Notably, GJA size and number of stitches were not associated with weight loss.
- Sutured revision of sleeve gastrectomy has been described in a case report and 5 patient case series. In the series, patients achieved a %TWL of 6.7% to 17.2% and mean %EWL of 33% at 1 year.[51]

SUMMARY

The current obesity pandemic has not been adequately addressed by previously available approaches. Endoscopic bariatric procedures may fill the treatment gap between medical therapy and bariatric surgery, while increasing the availability and palatability of weight loss interventions. The advent and widespread availability of a commercially available full-thickness suturing device and its application to the treatment of obesity has led to the creation of novel endoscopic techniques including ESG and TORe. Reports on ESG have been concentrated in expert centers, although its dissemination into clinical practice is accelerating. Several large series have demonstrated its efficacy, safety, and reproducibility, with improvements in metabolic diseases and a superior safety profile compared with bariatric surgery. Questions remain regarding durability owing to its recent implementation, although ESG may be repeated if necessary. Endoscopic revision of bariatric surgery, namely TORe, has level 1 evidence to support its efficacy and safety for the management of weight regain, as well as long-term follow-up data. As the bariatric surgery population continues to grow, procedures such as

TORe and LSG revision will play a primary role in the long-term management of these patients.

Clinicians interested in pursuing endoscopic suturing for bariatric procedures have several options for training including industry- and society-sponsored courses and preceptorships. To effectively deliver such therapies however, they should only be administered in the context of a comprehensive, multidisciplinary weight management program.

SUPPLEMENTARY DATA

Supplementary data related to this article can be found online at https://doi.org/10.1016/j.giec.2019.08.005.

REFERENCES

1. Ogden CL, Carroll MD, Kit BK, et al. Prevalence of childhood and adult obesity in the United States, 2011-2012. JAMA 2014;311(8):806–14.
2. Flegal KM, Kruszon-Moran D, Carroll MD, et al. Trends in obesity among adults in the United States, 2005 to 2014. JAMA 2016;315(21):2284–91.
3. Must A, Spadano J, Coakley EH, et al. The disease burden associated with overweight and obesity. J Am Med Assoc 1999;282(16):1523–9.
4. Gudzune KA, Doshi RS, Mehta AK, et al. Efficacy of commercial weight-loss programs: an updated systematic review. Ann Intern Med 2015;162(7):501–12.
5. Sacks FM, Bray GA, Carey VJ, et al. Comparison of weight-loss diets with different compositions of fat, protein, and carbohydrates. Obstet Gynecol Surv 2009;360(9):859–73.
6. Kumar RB, Aronne LJ. Efficacy comparison of medications approved for chronic weight management. Obesity (Silver Spring) 2015;23(Suppl 1):S4–7.
7. Avidor Y, Still CD, Brunner M, et al. Primary care and subspecialty management of morbid obesity: referral patterns for bariatric surgery. Surg Obes Relat Dis 2007;73(3):392–407.
8. Nguyen NT, Vu S, Kim E, et al. Trends in utilization of bariatric surgery, 2009–2012. Surg Endosc 2016;30(7):2723–7.
9. Fogel R, De Fogel J, Bonilla Y, et al. Clinical experience of transoral suturing for an endoluminal vertical gastroplasty: 1-year follow-up in 64 patients. Gastrointest Endosc 2008;68(1):51–8.
10. Brethauer SA, Chand B, Schauer PR, et al. Transoral gastric volume reduction for weight management: technique and feasibility in 18 patients. Surg Obes Relat Dis 2010;6(6):689–94.
11. Brethauer SA, Chand B, Schauer PR, et al. Transoral gastric volume reduction as intervention for weight management: 12-month follow-up of TRIM trial. Surg Obes Relat Dis 2012;118(3):296–303.
12. Stavropoulos SN, Modayil R, Friedel D. Current applications of endoscopic suturing. World J Gastrointest Endosc 2017;7(8):777–89.
13. Kumar N, Abu Dayyeh BK, Lopez-Nava Breviere G, et al. Endoscopic sutured gastroplasty: procedure evolution from first-in-man cases through current technique. Surg Endosc 2018;32(4):2159–64.
14. Abu Dayyeh BK, Rajan E, Gostout CJ. Endoscopic sleeve gastroplasty: a potential endoscopic alternative to surgical sleeve gastrectomy for treatment of obesity. Gastrointest Endosc 2013;78(3):530–5.

15. Lopez-Nava G, Galvao M, Bautista-Castaño I, et al. Endoscopic sleeve gastroplasty with 1-year follow-up: factors predictive of success. Endosc Int Open 2016;4(2):E222–7.
16. Abu Dayyeh BK, Acosta A, Camilleri M, et al. Endoscopic sleeve gastroplasty alters gastric physiology and induces loss of body weight in obese individuals. Clin Gastroenterol Hepatol 2017;15(1):37–43.e1.
17. Novikov AA, Afaneh C, Saumoy M, et al. Endoscopic sleeve gastroplasty, laparoscopic sleeve gastrectomy, and laparoscopic band for weight loss: how do they compare? J Gastrointest Surg 2018;22(2):267–73.
18. Sista F, Abruzzese V, Clementi M, et al. The effect of sleeve gastrectomy on GLP-1 secretion and gastric emptying: a prospective study. Surg Obes Relat Dis 2017; 13(1):7–14.
19. Sharaiha RZ, Kedia P, Kumta N, et al. Initial experience with endoscopic sleeve gastroplasty: technical success and reproducibility in the bariatric population. Endoscopy 2015;47(2):164–6.
20. Lopez-Nava G, Sharaiha RZ, Vargas EJ, et al. Endoscopic sleeve gastroplasty for obesity: a multicenter study of 248 patients with 24 months follow-up. Obes Surg 2017;27(10):2649–55.
21. Sartoretto A, Sui Z, Hill C, et al. Endoscopic sleeve gastroplasty (ESG) is a reproducible and effective endoscopic bariatric therapy suitable for widespread clinical adoption: a large, international multicenter study. Obes Surg 2018;28(7): 1812–21.
22. Sharaiha RZ, Kumta NA, Saumoy M, et al. Endoscopic sleeve gastroplasty significantly reduces body mass index and metabolic complications in obese patients. Clin Gastroenterol Hepatol 2017;15(4):504–10.
23. Alqahtani A, Al-Darwish A, Mahmoud A, et al. Short-term outcomes of endoscopic sleeve gastroplasty in 1000 consecutive patients. Gastrointest Endosc 2018;19(18):33363–7.
24. Lopez-Nava G, Galvão MP, Bautista-Castaño I, et al. Endoscopic sleeve gastroplasty for obesity treatment: two years of experience. Arq Bras Cir Dig 2017; 30(1):18–20.
25. Fayad L, Adam A, Schweitzer M, et al. Endoscopic sleeve gastroplasty versus laparoscopic sleeve gastrectomy: a case-matched study. Gastrointest Endosc 2019;89(4):782–8.
26. Graus Morales J, Crespo Pérez L, et al. Modified endoscopic gastroplasty for the treatment of obesity. Surg Endosc 2018;32(9):3936–42.
27. Hill C, El Zein M, Agnihotri A, et al. Endoscopic sleeve gastroplasty: the learning curve. Endosc Int Open 2017;5(9):E900–4.
28. Saumoy M, Schneider Y, Zhou XK, et al. A single-operator learning curve analysis for the endoscopic sleeve gastroplasty. Gastrointest Endosc 2018;87(2):442–7.
29. Brolin RE, Lin JM. Treatment of gastric leaks after Roux-en-Y gastric bypass: a paradigm shift. Surg Obes Relat Dis 2013;9(2):229–33.
30. McCormick JT, Papasavas PK, Caushaj PF, et al. Laparoscopic revision of failed open bariatric procedures. Surg Endosc Other Interv Tech 2003;3017(3):413–5.
31. Khaitan L, Van Sickle K, Gonzalez R, et al. Laparoscopic revision of bariatric procedures: is it feasible? Am Surg 2005;71(1):6–10.
32. Jirapinyo P, Dayyeh BKA, Thompson CC. Weight regain after Roux-en-Y gastric bypass has a large negative impact on the Bariatric Quality of Life Index. BMJ Open Gastroenterol 2017;4(1):e000153.
33. Shimizu H, Annaberdyev S, Motamarry I, et al. Revisional bariatric surgery for unsuccessful weight loss and complications. Obes Surg 2013;23(11):1766–73.

34. Khoursheed MA, Al-Bader IA, Al-Asfar FS, et al. Revision of failed bariatric procedures to Roux-en-Y gastric bypass (RYGB). Obes Surg 2011;21(8):1157–60.
35. Hedberg J, Gustavsson S, Sundbom M. Long-term follow-up in patients undergoing open gastric bypass as a revisional operation for previous failed restrictive procedures. Surg Obes Relat Dis 2012;8(6):696–701.
36. Buchwald H, Estok R, Fahrbach K, et al. Trends in mortality in bariatric surgery: a systematic review and meta-analysis. Surgery 2007;142(4):621–32.
37. Coakley BA, Deveney CW, Spight DH, et al. Revisional bariatric surgery for failed restrictive procedures. Surg Obes Relat Dis 2008;4(5):581–6.
38. Behrns KE, Smith CD, Kelly KA, et al. Reoperative bariatric surgery: lessons learned to improve patient selection and results. Ann Surg 1993;218(5):646–53.
39. Heneghan HM, Yimcharoen P, Brethauer SA, et al. Influence of pouch and stoma size on weight loss after gastric bypass. Surg Obes Relat Dis 2012;8(4):408–15.
40. Abu Dayyeh BK, Lautz DB, Thompson CC. Gastrojejunal stoma diameter predicts weight regain after Roux-en-Y gastric bypass. Clin Gastroenterol Hepatol 2011; 9(3):228–33.
41. Storm AC, Thompson CC. Endoscopic treatments following bariatric surgery. Gastrointest Endosc Clin North Am 2017;27(2):233–44.
42. Thompson CC, Slattery J, Bundga ME, et al. Peroral endoscopic reduction of dilated gastrojejunal anastomosis after Roux-en-Y gastric bypass: a possible new option for patients with weight regain. Surg Endosc Other Interv Tech 2006;20(11):1744–8.
43. Thompson CC, Chand B, Chen YK, et al. Endoscopic suturing for transoral outlet reduction increases weight loss after Roux-en-Y gastric bypass surgery. Gastroenterology 2013;145(1):129–37.e3.
44. Kumar N, Thompson CC. Comparison of a superficial suturing device with a full-thickness suturing device for transoral outlet reduction. Gastrointest Endosc 2014;79(6):984–9.
45. Patel LY, Lapin B, Brown CS, et al. Outcomes following 50 consecutive endoscopic gastrojejunal revisions for weight gain following Roux-en-Y gastric bypass: a comparison of endoscopic suturing techniques for stoma reduction. Surg Endosc 2017;31(6):2667–77.
46. Jirapinyo P, Slattery J, Ryan MB, et al. Evaluation of an endoscopic suturing device for transoral outlet reduction in patients with weight regain following Roux-en-Y gastric bypass. Endoscopy 2013;45(7):532–6.
47. Vargas EJ, Bazerbachi F, Rizk M, et al. Transoral outlet reduction with full thickness endoscopic suturing for weight regain after gastric bypass: a large multicenter international experience and meta-analysis. Surg Endosc 2018;32(1): 252–9.
48. Schulman AR, Kumar N, Thompson CC. Transoral outlet reduction: a comparison of purse-string with interrupted stitch technique. Gastrointest Endosc 2018;87(5): 1222–8.
49. Kumar N, Thompson CC. Transoral outlet reduction for weight regain after gastric bypass: long-term follow-up. Gastrointest Endosc 2016;83(4):776–9.
50. Jirapinyo P, Huseini M, Thompson CC. Five year outcomes following transoral outlet reduction (TORe) show effective and durable treatment of weight regain after ROUX-EN-Y gastric bypass. Gastroenterology 2017;152(5):S1308.
51. Eid G. Sleeve gastrectomy revision by endoluminal sleeve plication gastroplasty: a small pilot case series. Surg Endosc 2017;31(10):4252–5.

The Use of the OverStitch for Bariatric Weight Loss in Europe

Ravishankar Asokkumar, MBBS, MRCP[a,b,*],
Mohan Pappu Babu, MD[c], Inmaculada Bautista, MD, PhD[a],
Gontrand Lopez-Nava, MD, PhD[a]

KEYWORDS

- OverStitch • Endoscopic sleeve gastroplasty • Obesity treatment
- Bariatric endoscopy

KEY POINTS

- Endoscopic bariatric therapies are evolving to address the wide gap in obesity treatment.
- Endoscopic sleeve gastroplasty (ESG) is safe and effective in achieving weight loss and improvement in obesity-related comorbidities.
- The routine use of argon plasma coagulation to mark the sutures line before ESG may be avoided because it does not offer an additional advantage with suturing.
- Maintaining a proper orientation and adoption of the simplified technique may improve the operator efficiency and patient outcomes.

CASE DESCRIPTION

A 45-year-old, Mrs X, visited a clinic for the treatment of obesity. She weighed 90 kg, and the body mass index was 39.5 kg/m^2. She had a history of hypertension, diabetes mellitus, osteoarthropathy, and obstructive sleep apnea. Her symptoms were limiting her daily activity. She had enrolled in a medical weight loss program previously but had failed to lose weight. She had heard many unpleasant stories about bariatric surgery, including the risk of complications, development of reflux disease, dependence on supplements for long term, prolonged hospital stay, and high treatment cost. She is

Disclosure Statement: Dr G. Lopez-Nava is a consultant with Apollo Endosurgery and USGI Medical, USA. All other authors have no disclosure.
[a] Bariatric Endoscopy Unit, HM Sanchinarro University Hospital, Calle de Oña, 10, Madrid 28050, Spain; [b] Department of Gastroenterology and Hepatology, Singapore General Hospital, Singapore, Singapore; [c] Department of Internal Medicine, University of Arizona, Banner University Medical Center, 1625 North Campbell Avenue, Tucson, AZ 85719, USA
* Corresponding author. HM Sanchinarro University Hospital, Calle de Oña, 10, Madrid 28050, Spain.
E-mail address: ravishnkr03@gmail.com

motivated to lose weight and is requesting a less invasive effective treatment option so that she can get back to her preobese functional status.

INTRODUCTION

Several innovations and advancements have occurred in the field of interventional endoscopy in the past few decades, and the horizon for minimally invasive treatment has been vastly expanded. A new specialty of endoscopic surgery is evolving and is transforming the management of certain diseases, which were once solely treated by surgery.[1] It is now possible to resect early cancers, access the third space (submucosal) to remove submucosal tumors, perform myotomies, and create an artificial conduit between gastrointestinal lumen. More than ever, the basic and fundamental skill for surgery, which is tissue suturing, can now be performed endoscopically and can be utilized for myriad procedures, such as tissue approximation, closing iatrogenic and pathologic mucosal defects, fixing intraluminal devices, and achieving hemostasis.[2]

The concept of performing full-thickness suturing and approximating tissue through natural orifice without skin incision and without altering the anatomy has allowed exploring the option of recreating bariatric surgical procedures by endoscopy.[3] Since its first attempt in 2004, several modifications and improvement in the devices have occurred to enhance endoscopist experience and patient safety.[4] Currently, endoscopic gastroplasty techniques aimed at remodeling the stomach and reducing the gastric volume are emerging to become the mainstream bariatric procedures. The weight loss results observed so far is exciting and it has bridged the much-needed gap between pharmacotherapy and surgery.[5,6] Several platforms are available to perform endoscopic gastroplasty, and a few more are in development (**Fig. 1**).[7–11] The learning curve to master these techniques, however, can be steep.[12,13] This article describes the technique of endoscopic sleeve gastroplasty (ESG) and gastric volume reduction using the widely available OverStitch suturing device (Apollo Endosurgery, Austin, Texas) and provide guidance on the dos and don'ts for successful ESG.

KNOWING THE DEVICE
OverStitch Suturing Device

The suture system comprises the needle driver assembly, anchor exchange device, 2-0 polypropylene sutures, and accessories, such as the tissue helix and suture cinch. The device is compatible only with dual-channel endoscopes (GIF-2TH180 and GIF-2T160; Olympus, Center Valley, Pennsylvania). The needle driver assembly is mounted enface to the distal end of the scope, and the handle is attached to the proximal end, next to the working channel. The handle is squeezed to lock the needle body, and the anchor exchange device is advanced to engage and exchange the suture-anchor assembly for performing the stitching operations (**Fig. 2**). The device, however, has few limitations: (1) only compatible with dual channel endoscope, which is not widely available; (2) the endoscope is stiff and less maneuverable; (3) the field of vision gets impaired when the device is mounted; and (4) the ability to suction decreases with the presence of accessories in the working channel. To overcome these limitations, a newer device has been made available.

OverStitch Sx Device

The single-channel endoscopic suturing system (Overstitch Sx, Apollo Endosurgery, Austin, TX) can be mounted on most endoscopes with a diameter ranging from 8.8 mm to 9.8 mm. It has an external catheter sheath, which has 2 separate working

Procedure	Manufacturer	Device	Technique
Endoscopic Sleeve Gastroplasty (ESG)	Apollo Endosurgery, USA	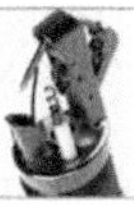	Full-thickness continuous suturing
Primary Obesity Surgery Endoluminal (POSE)	USGI Medical, USA	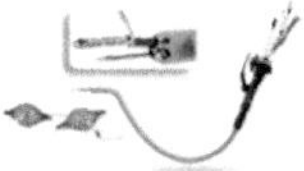	Tissue plication using snowshoe suture anchors
Endomina Triangulation Platform	EndoTools Therapeutics, Belgium	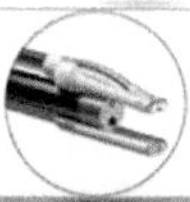	Transmural serosa-to-serosa apposition
Articulating Circular Stapling device (ACE)	Boston Scientific, USA	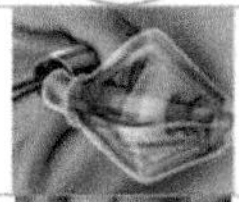	360° full-thickness stapling
Endozip	Nitinotes Surgical, Israel	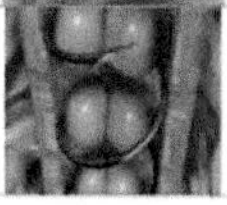	Automated full-thickness suturing

Fig. 1. Endoscopic gastroplasty techniques and devices. (*Adapted from* Huberty V, Ibrahim M, Hiernaux M, Chau A, Dugardeyn S, Deviere J. Safety and feasibility of an endoluminalsuturing device for endoscopic gastric reduction (with video). Gastrointestinal Endoscopy. 2017;85(4):833-837; and Verlaan T, Paulus GF, Mathus- Vliegen EMH, Veldhuyzen EAML, Conchillo JM, Bouvy ND, et al. Endoscopic gastric volume reduction with a novel articulating plication device is safe and effective in the treatment of obesity (with video). Gastrointestinal Endoscopy. 2015;81(2):312-320; and *Courtesy of* Apollo Endosurgery, Inc., Austin, TX; USGI Medical, San Clemente, CA; Endo Tools Therapeutics, Gosselies, Belgium; Boston Scientific, Inc., Marlborough, MA; and Nitinotes Surgical, Ltd., Caesarea, Israel, with permission.)

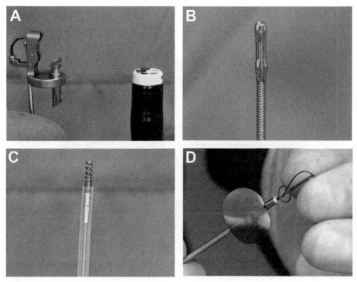

Fig. 2. (*A*) The needle driver assembly, (*B*) anchor exchange device, (*C*) tissue helix, and (*D*) cinch catheter.

channels independent of the scope channel and can be used to operate the Over-Stitch accessories (anchor exchange, tissue helix, and suture cinch). The needle driver assembly is fixed at the side of the distal scope end and does not interfere with the field of view. The longer length of the endcap with the needle driver assembly enables capturing a large amount of tissue with the full-thickness bites (**Fig. 3**).

ENDOSCOPIC SLEEVE GASTROPLASTY

The technique of ESG has undergone several changes and technical refinement since its introduction. The first few cases were performed in retroflexion to target the fundus first and then progressed distally to antrum. This technique is, however, cumbersome, time-consuming, and seldom followed.[14] The suturing is now started from the distal stomach and progressed proximally involving the greater curvature and sparing both the fundus and antrum. Similarly, a variety of stitch patterns and sequences were studied to improve the procedure outcome and endoscopist efficiency. In the initial reports, more than 23 to 28 sutures were used to achieve desired gastric volume reduction. With progressive evolution, there is a trend to using fewer sutures to perform ESG. To date, the application of interrupted suture, continuous suture, M pattern, Z pattern, triangular, and U-shaped pattern have all been described.[15] But no 1 suture pattern is superior in achieving better outcomes. Likewise, the need for preprocedure Argon plasma coagulation (APC) marking, number of sutures required, bites per stitch, placement of reinforcement sutures, and tightness of cinching are still being debated.

The cardinal goal of ESG is to shorten and narrow the stomach and alter the gastric motility without increasing the risk of complications and cost with the procedure. By inducing alteration in gastric physiology, a durable weight loss may be achieved even after the loss of suture in the future.

HOW THE AUTHORS DO ENDOSCOPIC SLEEVE GASTROPLASTY

The authors have simplified the technique of ESG based on the lessons learned from prior experience and understanding of the principles behind surgical suturing techniques. With ESG, the authors aim to create multiple internal segmentation to reduce

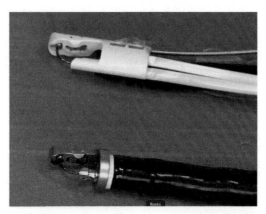

Fig. 3. The conventional suturing device (below) mounted on the distal end of a double channel endoscope and the new suturing device (above) suitable for most single-channel scopes. The needle driver assembly of a single-channel scope is longer (2 cm) than the conventional device (1.5 cm) and can capture a large amount of tissue.

the size of the stomach and form pockets to promote stasis of food and induce satiation.

The authors perform the procedure with the patient under general anesthesia and in left lateral position. An overtube is inserted and the stomach inspected for the presence of adverse pathology before performing gastroplasty.[4] Antibiotics are administered before ESG and use CO_2 insufflation and water jet function. The correct orientation of the stomach is maintained throughout the procedure to guide suturing. The authors do not use APC to mark the suture lines before ESG for 2 reasons. First, the stomach is dynamic, and the APC lines move after each suture plication, making it a less reliable marker for subsequent sutures. Second, the mucosal bleeding after each full-thickness bites may make the APC markings less visible. A U-shaped suture pattern is performed, comprising 8 full-thickness suture bites (**Fig. 4**). This pattern foreshortens the stomach and reduces the length by more than 40% and also narrows the gastric lumen.[16] The authors ensure that the suture travels in 1 direction throughout the procedure and do not routinely perform additional reinforcement sutures.

The authors capture the tissue using the helix device and rotate the cap clockwise 3 times to anchor it and do not use suction alone to capture the tissue inside the needle driver because this may result in superficial suture bites. To achieve full-thickness bites consistently, the tissue obtained by the helix is placed perpendicular to the needle driver. The authors always start at the anterior wall, 1-cm proximal to incisura, continue to traverse through the greater curvature to the posterior wall, and repeat the pattern in reverse before the method of performing continuous suture is cinched to form a plication (**Fig. 5**). This method of performing continuous suture involving the greater curve may affect the receptive and adaptive relaxation of the gastric body. The antrum also is not included in the suture because the propulsion and mixing function of the antral pump may usually result in early suture loss. The authors advocate applying intermittent and incremental tension to tighten the suture while cinching because this brings the walls of the stomach together to form a sleeve. The second suture is started 1 cm to 2 cm proximal to the first suture plication to create a pocket for food stasis between the sutures. The authors follow these steps and perform 4 to 5 suture plications in the proximal gastric body. The fundus is spared. It functions as a small pouch and involving the thin fundal wall (2.6 mm) in the transmural suture may only increase the risk of vascular and adjacent organ injury.[16] The authors do not

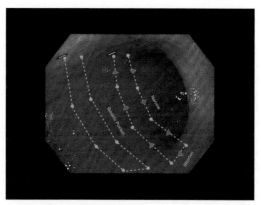

Fig. 4. U-shaped suture pattern starting and ending on the same side of the stomach. This pattern foreshortens and narrows the gastric lumen significantly.

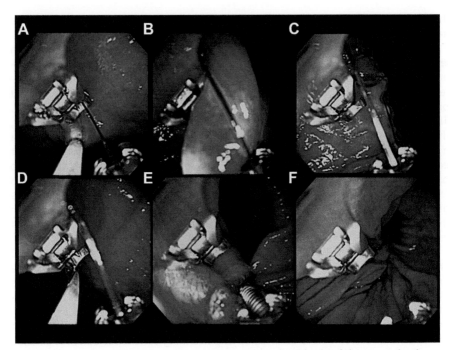

Fig. 5. Endoscopic creation of a suture plication at the distal body of the stomach. The authors (*A*) capture the tissue using the helix at the anterior wall of the stomach; (*B*) traction and position it perpendicular to the needle driver to take a full-thickness bite; (*C*) perform a continuous suture and traverse through the greater curvature of the stomach; (*D*) reach the posterior wall and include that in the suture and repeat the pattern in reverse until the anterior wall is reached again; (*E*) apply gentle intermittent tension on the suture to bring together the opposing walls to form a sleeve (not applying forceful traction to avoid suture breakage); and (*F*) successful narrowing of the lumen after cinching.

routinely advance the scope to the pylorus or duodenum after ESG because overdistention and inadvertent manipulation may loosen the sutures.

WEIGHT-LOSS COMPARISON

The recommended absolute threshold for a primary bariatric therapy includes achieving greater than 25% excess weight loss (EWL) or greater than 10% total body weight loss (TBWL) at 12 months and a mean percentage EWL difference of 15% compared with the control group. Several studies have reported the outcomes with ESG since its first description in 2013. There was considerable variation in the scales, however, used for reporting weight loss outcomes, and some studies had overlapping patients.

The authors identified 6 good-quality studies (n 5, 1600) on ESG. The percent (%) TBWL and %EWL at 6 months and 12 months were 15.6% and 17.5%, and 59.7% and 64.1%, respectively.[12,17–21] The overall adverse event rate was 3.2% (**Table 1**). Lopez-Nava and colleagues[22] showed at 24 months the %TBWL was 18.6%. Only 1 study to date (presented in abstract form) reported the long-term weight loss results after ESG. It showed at 5 years that the weight loss achieved was 18.7 kg and the % TBWL was 14.5%.[23] Similarly, Sharaiha and colleagues[24] and Alqahtani and colleagues[17] have reported improvement in diabetes mellitus, hypertension, and

Table 1
Weight loss outcomes with endoscopic sleeve gastroplasty

Author	Study Design	Setting	Patients (n)	Body Mass Index (SD), kg/m^2	Percent Total Body Weight Loss (SD)	Length of Stay
Alqahtani et al,[17] 2019	Prospective	Single center	1000	33.3 (4.5)	15.5 (7.7)	1–2 d
Fayad et al,[18] 2019	Retrospective	Single center	58	41.5 (8.2)	21.3 (6.6)	NR
Graus Morales et al,[19] 2018	Retrospective	Single center	148	35.1 (5.5)	17.5 (7.6)	1–2 d
Sartoretto et al,[20] 2018	Retrospective	Multi-center	112	37.9 (6.7)	14.9 (6.1)	1 d
Saumoy et al,[12] 2018	Prospective	Single center	128	38.9 (6.9)	15.8 (9.5)	NR
Lopez-Nava et al,[21] 2017	Prospective	Single center	154	38.3 (5.5)	18.2 (10.1)	1 d

Abbreviation: NR, not reported.

hyperlipidemia after ESG. There are few data comparing the outcome of ESG with its surgical counterpart, the laparoscopic sleeve gastrectomy (LSG).

A retrospective case-matched study showed the %TBWL at 6 months with LSG was significantly more compared with ESG (23.6% vs 17.1%; *P*<.01). But the adverse event rate was higher with LSG (16.9% vs 5.2%; *P*<.05) with an increased incidence of new-onset gastroesophageal reflux disease (GERD) (14.5% vs1.9%).[25] To better compare, the authors identified 7 studies (n = 2179), published after 2013 that reported the outcome of LSG at 12 months (**Table 2**). The authors found the %TWBL and %EWL at 12 months were 30.5% and 69.3%, respectively. The risk of adverse events was 11.8%, and the rate of GERD was 5.8%.[26–32]

Table 2
Weight loss outcomes with laparoscopic sleeve gastroplasty

Author	Study Design	Setting	Patients (n)	Body Mass index (SD), kg/m^2	Percent Excell Weight Loss (SD)	Length of Stay
El-Matbouly et al,[26] 2018	Retrospective	Single center	91	48 (7.5)	49.5 (25.8)	2–4 d
Talebpour et al,[27] 2018	Randomized	Single center	35	44.6 (3.5)	65.4 (16.5)	5–7 d
Wang et al,[28] 2016	Retrospective	Single center	70	40.8 (5.9)	77.1 (13.0)	NR
Alvarenga et al,[29] 2016	Retrospective	Multi-center	1020	43.4 (5.8)	86 (22.3)	2–5 d
Lemaître et al,[30] 2016	Retrospective	Single center	494	47.8 (7.8)	64 (23.5)	3–21 d
Golomb et al,[31] 2015	Retrospective	Single center	241	41.9 (6.7)	76.8	NR
Zachariah et al,[32] 2013	Retrospective	Single center	228	37.4 (4.7)	72.4 (16)	1–2 d

Abbreviation: NR, not reported.

Based on the reported evidence, ESG seems a safe and effective treatment of obesity with a low complication rate. It may become an attractive and patient preferred treatment option because of its minimal invasiveness, shorter length of stay, and lower procedure cost.

COMPLICATIONS WITH ENDOSCOPIC SUTURING AND GASTROPLASTY—HOW TO AVOID THEM

Although safe, complications sometimes can occur after endoscopic suturing and gastroplasty.[17–22,33–35] The overall serious adverse event rate was 1.1% (**Table 3**). A majority of them were managed conservatively or by endoscopy. The authors describe some of the technical steps and safety measures that could be used during the procedure to prevent complications.

During Insertion

The needle driver assembly is made of stainless steel and protrudes beyond the distal flexible end of the scope. While introducing through the narrow upper esophageal sphincter, the metallic end may lacerate the mucosa and cause bleeding. Similarly, insertion of the endoscope with the needle driver in the open position exposes the sharp end of the needle, and, additionally, the extended elbow of the needle may stretch and tear the esophageal mucosa. This easily can be prevented by using the recommended overtube. The authors suggest advancing the scope holding the overtube for a controlled scope insertion (**Fig. 6**).

During Suturing

Several problems could be encountered during the gastroplasty procedure. They can be related to the technique, device, or accessories.

Accidental suture tag release

The critical learning in endoscopic suturing is to become familiar and effortless with the steps of suture transfer between the needle driver and the anchor exchange catheter because these steps are performed multiple times to create a full-thickness continuous suture. Locking the needle driver with the anchor exchange catheter outside the channel may result in damaging the suturing system (**Fig. 7**).

During the learning phase, the suture tag can be accidently released in the stomach before completing the desired suture pattern, resulting in the need for additional sutures materials, which can be expensive (**Fig. 8**). Also, the suture tag can be released

Table 3	
Risk of serious adverse events after ESG from available studies (n = 1612)	
Serious Adverse Events	**Reported Occurrences (%)**
Mortality	0 (0)
Bleeding requiring transfusion/intervention	6 (0.4)
Gall bladder capture requiring surgery	2 (0.1)
Intra-abdominal collection	7 (0.4)
Perforation	1 (0.06)
Pneumothorax/pneumoperitoneum	1 (0.06)
Pulmonary embolism	1 (0.06)
ESG reversal	3 (0.2)

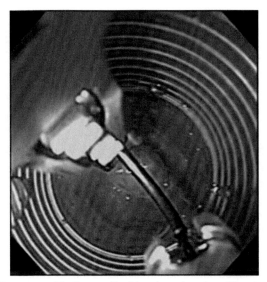

Fig. 6. Introduce the scope with the needle driver in a closed position to avoid injury to the oropharynx and the esophagus. Use an overtube to protect the mucosa and allow easy scope navigation.

inadvertently inside the scope channel, resulting in damage to the scope. Gaining competence in the basic steps is mandatory before embarking to endoscopic suturing.

Suture loop formation
The OverSitch device uses a 2-0 monofilament prolene suture, which can easily pass through tissue without inciting an inflammatory reaction. It lacks elasticity and memory, however, and has poor knot security. Thus, for successful gastroplasty, it is

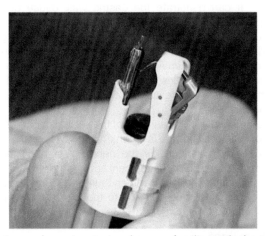

Fig. 7. Before starting endoscopic suturing, become familiar with the task of exchanging the suture between the needle driver and anchor exchange catheter. Attempting to close the needle driver with anchor exchange catheter outside the channel may damage the device.

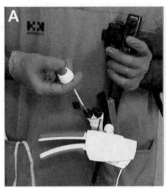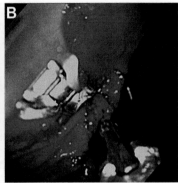

Fig. 8. (*A*) Accidental release of suture tag before completion of the desired U- shaped suture pattern. (*B*) The suture tag can be seen immediately after the first bite. Additional suture would be required to create the sleeve.

essential to approximate the opposing wall with minimum tension. To achieve this, the authors follow a U-shaped suture pattern similar to the horizontal mattress sutures in surgery, where the suture travels in 1 direction and enters and exits on the same side. Changing the direction of the suture in between the full-thickness bites and forming alpha loops increase the elasticity and cause suture breakage and incomplete tissue approximation (**Fig. 9**).

Tissue laceration and entrapment of adjacent organs

Tissue laceration can occur from the helix device or the metallic tip of the needle drive assembly resulting in bleeding. The tissue, when pulled with a superficially embedded helix, can result in disanchoring and mucosal injury. Similarly, tissue traction when the metallic needle driver assembly is in contact with the gastric wall can cause stripping of the superficial gastric mucosa and oozing (**Fig. 10**).

Care must be taken when using the tissue helix device. When drilled deeper with excessive pressure, it can penetrate the gastric wall, cause pneumoperitoneum/leak, and also trap the adjacent structures. The authors experienced a case of gall bladder laceration and entrapment after ESG, which required surgical release and removal of the gallbladder (**Fig. 11**). The authors believe deep drilling of the mucosa with helix and involving the proximal antrum in the ESG may have resulted in this adverse event. Peng and colleagues,[36] in their laparoscopy-assisted ESG, showed 4 rotations of the helix device lead to sufficient entrapment of gastric mucosa without penetrating the abdominal cavity.

The authors recommend 3 clockwise turns of the helix to capture the tissue. The authors suggest positioning the scope a few centimeters away from the target area and pulling the helix with the tissue inside the needle assembly, thereby preventing mucosal pressure injury and displacing adjacent structures from the path of the needle track (see **Fig. 10**). Whenever resistance is encountered during traction, the authors rotate the helix anticlockwise once or twice to reduce the tissue bulk or remove it and choose a different site for suturing.

Frayed suture and breakage

Suture damage, fracturing, and gaping of the plication may prolong the procedure time and require additional suturing, which can be expensive. The suture damage and fracturing mainly occur during cinching. When excessive tension is applied on

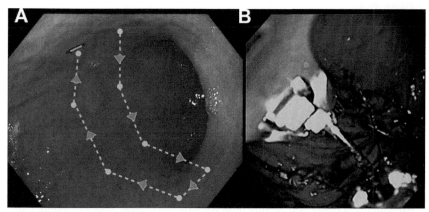

Fig. 9. Loop formation may result in inadequate tissue apposition or may result in the cutting of suture. (*A*) An ideal suture should preferentially traverse in one direction without the formation of loops. (*B*) The crossing of sutures may result in incomplete convergence of tissue.

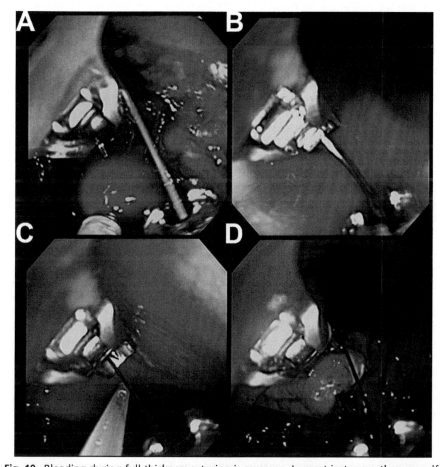

Fig. 10. Bleeding during full-thickness suturing is common. In most instances, they are self-limiting and can be managed conservatively. Bleeding can be either from (*A*) the tissue drilling using the helix device or (*B*) the pressure exerted by the metallic tip of the needle driver assemble. To minimize bleeding, (*C*) approach the target area from a distance and avoid mucosal contact with the metallic tip and (*D*) avoid superficial helix placement, which can result in tissue chipping.

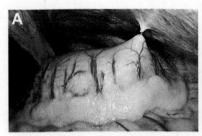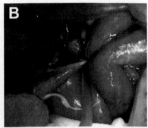

Fig. 11. Inadvertent capture of an adjacent structure may occur during ESG. (*A*) The pressure exerted on the helix device and deeper drilling of the device map penetrate the gastric wall into the abdominal cavity and capture adjacent structures. Laparoscopy monitored endoscopic gastroplasty suggests that rotatin the helix device beyond 4 turns may lead to deeper penetration. (*B*) Gallbladder laceration and entrapment in full-thickness suture resulting in biliary peritonitis. Surgery was required to release and remove the gallbladder. (**Fig. 11**A, *From* Peng L, Li X, Zhang G. Guidance for full-thickness suturing in endoscopic sleeve gastroplasty - preliminary exploration using laparoscopy. Endoscopy. 2019 Mar;51(3):E61-E62. https://doi.org/10.1055/a-0820-1294. Epub 2019 Jan 11; with permission.)

the suture, exceeding its elasticity, the suture fibers start to separate and become thin, resulting in breakage before cinching.

Similarly, gaping of sutures may occur during the procedure when the opposing tissues are prematurely cinched or may be observed during follow-up in patients who have a very tight sleeve with increased intragastric pressure and are not compliant with dietary instruction (**Fig. 12**). The authors recommend applying slow, graded, intermittent traction to get all the gastric walls together under visual guidance. The authors abort applying traction when suture wearing out is observed. The authors suggest not creating a tight sleeve and ensuring the endoscope can easily traverse through the sleeve to the duodenum. In the situation of gaping or disconnection of the sleeve, the authors perform a touch-up revision of ESG by placing 1 or 2 sutures to maintain continuity. They are technically easier than the initial procedure.

Cinch device malfunction

Cinch device malfunction, although infrequent, can be a challenging complication to manage. The cinching and suture cutting involves 3 process—(1) locking the suture using the cinch plug, (2) engaging the suture cutter, and (3) activating the cutter and slicing the suture. When excessive suture tension is applied during cinching, the spring inside the handle of the cinch device may fracture and malfunction and may fail to engage and activate the suture cutter. The cinch with the trapped and uncut suture cannot be removed from the endoscope channel. In such situations, the cinch handle needs to be dismantled, and the central stiff metallic wire leading to the cutting system should be captured and pulled manually to activate it and severe the suture (**Fig. 13**). To avoid encountering such technical difficulties, the authors suggest releasing the suture tension slightly just before squeezing the cinch handle.

During Withdrawal

Inadvertent gastric and esophageal laceration may occur if the scope is withdrawn without locking the needle driver assembly. The authors recommend ensuring the needle driver system is free of sutures and gastric tissue. The authors lock the device and gently withdraw the scope inside over tube and remove the scope together with the overtube.

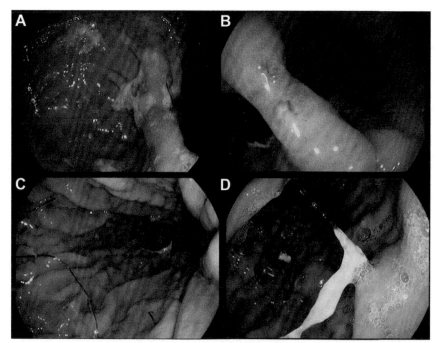

Fig. 12. (*A, B*) Follow-up endoscopy performed at 1-year showed intact mucosal bridging and maintenance of narrow gastric lumen. (*C, D*) In some cases, where the weight loss plateaus, suture gaping can be observed. This can be managed efficiently by doing touch-up suturing to reinforce the sleeve contour. This is easier and quicker than the initial gastroplasty.

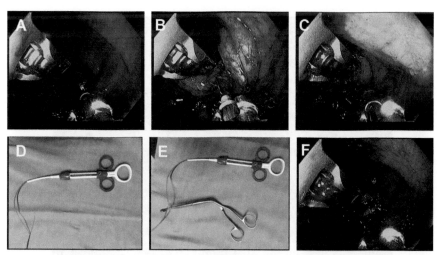

Fig. 13. Cinch breakage and failure is the most challenging problem to troubleshoot. (*A*) Cinch catheter introduced over the suture to complete the plication. (*B*) The plug of the cinch has engaged the suture inside the catheter but fails to activate the cutting mechanism. (*C*) The plug of the cinch cannot be reopened once engaged firmly inside the catheter. (*D*) Forceful closure of the cinch handle, in an attempt to cut the suture, may result in fracturing of the lever within the handle. (*E*) In such instances, the handle needs to be cut open, and the long metallic wire/rod connected to the cutting system at the distal end should be manually trapped and pulled to release the plug. (*F*) Successful cinching and release of the plug.

EXTENDED APPLICATION IN ENDOBARIATRICS
Postsurgical Weight Regain

Weight regain and recurrence of comorbidity after bariatric surgery (Roux-en-Y gastric bypass) area is a significant problem and affect approximately one-third of patients. The dilation of gastrojejunal (GJ) anastomosis (>10 mm) is an independent predictive factor for weight regain after surgery. Traditionally, this was addressed by refashioning of the GJ anastomosis by surgery, which can be complicated and associated with significant morbidity. With the availability of endoscopic suturing, transoral reduction of the anastomotic outlet can be performed safely as a short-stay procedure with no major complications (**Fig. 14**).[37,38] Several suture patterns like the interrupted suture, purse-string suture, U-shaped pattern, and figure-of-8 pattern have been described with similar efficacy. A recent meta-analysis (n = 330) showed the pooled weight loss at 12 months was 8.4 kg (95% CI 6.5–10.3) with no serious adverse events.[39]

Gastroesophageal Reflux Disease

Endoscopic suturing can be extended to treat proton pump inhibitor (PPI) refractory or intolerant GERD and postsurgical reflux disease. An increasing number of patients develop new-onset GERD after sleeve gastrectomy and may not be good candidates for fundoplication procedures. Han and colleagues,[40] in a pilot study on 10 patients, showed endoscopic suturing is feasible and safe to treat obesity. In their short-term follow-up, they showed significant improvement in GERD-health related quality of life scores. The durability of the sutures, however, was inadequate. To overcome this, the same group modified the technique to combine mucosal ablation using APC along the lesser curvature of the cardia, immediately below the gastroesophageal junction, followed by endoscopic suturing to create a tightened tissue valve to prevent

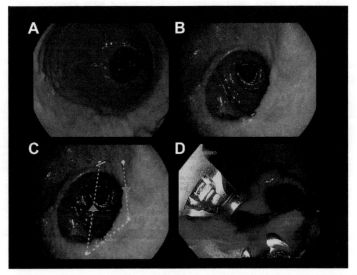

Fig. 14. Transoral endoscopic outlet reduction to manage post–Roux-en-Y gastric bypass weight regain. (A) A grossly dilated gastric pouch can be observed, (B) the GJ anastomosis is widely opened and approximately 3 cm to 4 cm in size, (C) continuous suture pattern used to decrease the size of the GJ anastomosis (APC also can be applied to freshen the mucosa before suturing), and (D) The size of the GJ is significantly reduced. Additional continuous sutures in the distal gastric pouch will also reduce the size of the dilated pouch.

reflux (mucosal ablation and suturing at the esophagogastric junction procedure). At 4 months, 59% were off PPI, and 14% showed a reduction in PPI dose with no early or late complications.[41]

CLINICAL CASE OUTCOME

Mrs X opted for ESG and was adherent to the multidisciplinary follow-up program. During the review at 1-year, she has lost 18 kg, and the %TBWL was 20%. The dosage of her diabetes medication has decreased by 50% and she is not on any antihypertensive drugs or nocturnal continuous positive airway pressure. Her quality of life has improved, and she is more productive at work than before after the weight loss. She is still on follow-up and is motivated to maintain weight loss.

SUMMARY

Interventional endoscopists are fortunate to have witnessed an enormous evolution in their field. It is time for endoscopists and surgeons to collaborate and expand the specialty of minimally invasive endoscopic surgery. The road to the future is exciting, and, with emerging innovations and training, the course of many diseases can be altered and an impact made on the lives of many patients. ESG is ready for prime time and will fill the gap in the obesity treatment paradigm.

REFERENCES

1. Chang KJ. Endoscopic foregut surgery and interventions: The future is now. The state-of-the-art and my personal journey. World J Gastroenterol 2019;25(1):1–41.
2. Stavropoulos SN, Modayil R, Friedel D. Current applications of endoscopic suturing. World J Gastrointest Endosc 2015;7(8):777–89.
3. Abu Dayyeh BK, Rajan E, Gostout CJ. Endoscopic sleeve gastroplasty: a potential endoscopic alternative to surgical sleeve gastrectomy for treatment of obesity. Gastrointest Endosc 2013;78(3):530–5.
4. Fogel R, De Fogel J, Bonilla Y, et al. Clinical experience of transoral suturing for an endoluminal vertical gastroplasty: 1-year follow-up in 64 patients. Gastrointest Endosc 2008;68(1):51–8.
5. Khan Z, Khan MA, Hajifathalian K, et al. Efficacy of endoscopic interventions for the management of obesity: a meta-analysis to compare endoscopic sleeve gastroplasty, AspireAssist, and primary obesity surgery endolumenal. Obes Surg 2019;29(7):2287–98.
6. Jirapinyo P, Thompson CC. Endoscopic bariatric and metabolic therapies: surgical analogues and mechanisms of action. Clin Gastroenterol Hepatol 2017;15(5):619–30.
7. Espinos JC, Turro R, Mata A, et al. Early experience with the Incisionless Operating Platform (IOP) for the treatment of obesity: The Primary Obesity Surgery Endolumenal (POSE) procedure. Obes Surg 2013;23(9):1375–83.
8. Lopez-Nava G, Bautista-Castano I, Jimenez A, et al. The Primary Obesity Surgery Endolumenal (POSE) procedure: one-year patient weight loss and safety outcomes. Surg Obes Relat Dis 2015;11(4):861–5.
9. Huberty V, Ibrahim M, Hiernaux M, et al. Safety and feasibility of an endoluminal-suturing device for endoscopic gastric reduction (with video). Gastrointest Endosc 2017;85(4):833–7.

10. Verlaan T, Paulus GF, Mathus- Vliegen EMH, et al. Endoscopic gastric volume reduction with a novel articulating plication device is safe and effective in the treatment of obesity (with video). Gastrointest Endosc 2015;81(2):312–20.

11. Lopez-Nava G, Asokkumar R, Bautista-Castaño I. First in human results of Endozip, A novel suturing bariatric endoscopy procedure. Gastrointest Endosc 2019;89(6):AB270.

12. Saumoy M, Schneider Y, Zhou XK, et al. A single-operator learning curve analysis for the endoscopic sleeve gastroplasty. Gastrointest Endosc 2018;87(2):442–7.

13. Hill C, El Zein M, Agnihotri A, et al. Endoscopic sleeve gastroplasty: the learning curve. Endosc Int Open 2017;5(9):E900–4.

14. Kumar N, Abu Dayyeh BK, Lopez-Nava G, et al. Endoscopic sutured gastroplasty: procedure evolution from first-in-man cases through current technique. Surg Endosc 2018;32(4):2159–64.

15. Jain D, Bhandari BS, Arora A, et al. Endoscopic sleeve gastroplasty - a new tool to manage obesity. Clin Endosc 2017;50(6):552–61.

16. James TW, McGowan CE. The descending gastric fundus in endoscopic sleeve gastroplasty: implications for procedural technique and adverse events. VideoGIE 2019;4(6):254–5.

17. Alqahtani A, Al-Darwish A, Mahmoud AE, et al. Short-term outcomes of endoscopic sleeve gastroplasty in 1000 consecutive patients. Gastrointest Endosc 2019;89(6):1132–8.

18. Fayad L, Cheskin LJ, Adam A, et al. Endoscopic sleeve gastroplasty versus intragastric balloon insertion: efficacy, durability, and safety. Endoscopy 2019;51(6):532–9.

19. Graus Morales J, Crespo Pérez L, Marques A, et al. Modified endoscopic gastroplasty for the treatment of obesity. Surg Endosc 2018;32(9):3936–42.

20. Sartoretto A, Sui Z, Hill C, et al. Endoscopic sleeve gastroplasty (ESG) is a reproducible and effective endoscopic bariatric therapy suitable for widespread clinical adoption: a large, international multicenter study. Obes Surg 2018;28(7):1812–21.

21. Lopez-Nava G, Galvão MP, Bautista-Castaño I, et al. Endoscopic sleeve gastroplasty for obesity treatment: two years of experience. Arq Bras Cir Dig 2017;30(1):18–20.

22. Lopez-Nava G, Sharaiha RZ, Vargas EJ, et al. Endoscopic sleeve gastroplasty for obesity: a multicenter study of 248 patients with 24 months follow-up. Obes Surg 2017;27(10):2649–55.

23. Kaveh H, Bryan A, Qais MD, et al. Long term follow up and outcome after endoscopic sleeve gastroplasty for treatment of obesity (5 year data). Gastrointest Endosc 2019;89(6):AB58.

24. Sharaiha RZ, Kumta NA, Saumoy M, et al. Endoscopic sleeve gastroplasty significantly reduces body mass index and metabolic complications in obese patients. Clin Gastroenterol Hepatol 2017;15(4):504–10.

25. Fayad L, Adam A, Schweitzer M, et al. Endoscopic sleeve gastroplasty versus laparoscopic sleeve gastrectomy: a case-matched study. Gastrointest Endosc 2019;89(4):782–8.

26. El-Matbouly MA, Khidir N, Touny HA, et al. A 5-year follow-up study of laparoscopic sleeve gastrectomy among morbidly obese adolescents: does it improve body image and prevent and treat diabetes? Obes Surg 2018;28(2):513–9.

27. Talebpour M, Sadid D, Talebpour A, et al. Comparison of short-term effectiveness and postoperative complications: laparoscopic gastric plication vs laparoscopic sleeve gastrectomy. Obes Surg 2018;28(4):996–1001.

28. Wang X, Chang XS, Gao L, et al. Effectiveness of laparoscopic sleeve gastrectomy for weight loss and obesity-associated co-morbidities: a 3-year outcome from Mainland Chinese patients. Surg Obes Relat Dis 2016;12(7):1305–11.

29. Alvarenga ES, Lo Menzo E, Szomstein S, et al. Safety and efficacy of 1020 consecutive laparoscopic sleeve gastrectomies performed as a primary treatment modality for morbid obesity. A single-center experience from the metabolic and bariatric surgical accreditation quality and improvement program. Surg Endosc 2016;30(7):2673–8.

30. Lemaître F, Léger P, Nedelcu M, et al. Laparoscopic sleeve gastrectomy in the South Pacific. Retrospective evaluation of 510 patients in a single institution. Int J Surg 2016;30:1–6.

31. Golomb I, Ben David M, Glass A, et al. Long-term metabolic effects of laparoscopic sleeve gastrectomy. JAMA Surg 2015;150(11):1051–7.

32. Zachariah SK, Chang PC, Ooi AS, et al. Laparoscopic sleeve gastrectomy for morbid obesity: 5 years experience from an Asian center of excellence. Obes Surg 2013;23(7):939–46.

33. Pyda P, Sowier A, Sowier S, et al. Initial experience with endoscopic sleeve gastroplasty in Poland. Pol Przegl Chir 2018;90(4):35–40.

34. James TW, Sheikh SZ, McGowan CE. Perigastric abscess as a delayed adverse event in endoscopic sleeve gastroplasty. Gastrointest Endosc 2019;89(4):890–1.

35. Lopez-Nava G, Asokkumar R, Ielpo B, et al. Biliary peritonitis after endoscopic sutured gastroplasty for morbid obesity (with video). Gastrointest Endosc 2019. [Epub ahead of print].

36. Peng L, Li X, Zhang G. Guidance for full-thickness suturing in endoscopic sleeve gastroplasty - preliminary exploration using laparoscopy. Send Endosc 2019; 51(3):E61–2.

37. Fayad L, Schweitzer M, Raad M. A real-world, insurance-based algorithm using the two-fold running suture technique for transoral outlet reduction for weight regain and dumping syndrome after roux-en-Y gastric bypass. Obes Surg 2019; 29(7):2225–32.

38. Jirapinyo P, Kröner PT, Thompson CC. Purse-string transoral outlet reduction (TORe) is effective at inducing weight loss and improvement in metabolic comorbidities after Roux-en-Y gastric bypass. Endoscopy 2018;50(4):371–7.

39. Vargas EJ, Bazerbachi F, Rizk M, et al. Transoral outlet reduction with full thickness endoscopic suturing for weight regain after gastric bypass: a large multicenter international experience and meta-analysis. Surg Endosc 2018;32(1): 252–9.

40. Han J, Chin M, Fortinsky KJ, et al. Endoscopic augmentation of gastroesophageal junction using a full-thickness endoscopic suturing device. Endosc Int Open 2018;6(9):E1120–5.

41. Kyle JF, Toshitaka S, Matt AC, et al. Mucosal ablation and suturing at the esophagigastric junction (MASE): a novel procedure for the management of patients with gastroesophageal reflux disease. Gastrointest Endosc 2018;87(6):AB552.

The Use of the Overstitch to Close Perforations and Fistulas

Phillip S. Ge, MD[a], Christopher C. Thompson, MD, MSc[b],*

KEYWORDS

- Endoscopic suturing • Fistula • Leak • Overstitch • Perforation

KEY POINTS

- Fundamental principles of perforation, leak, and fistula management include identification of the site of disruption, drainage of any leaked contents, and controlling the flow of luminal contents with either diversion or closure.
- Endoscopic suturing may be superior to endoclips in the management of perforations, due to the ability of the Overstitch device to achieve full-thickness "surgical-quality" suturing and create an airtight closure.
- A full-thickness running suture pattern (compared with interrupted, horizontal mattress, and pursestring patterns) produces the most robust perforation closure, with highest leak pressure, and can be completed faster than other suturing patterns.
- Although successful closure of leaks and fistulas using endoscopic suturing has been described in the literature, recurrence is common and additional therapy with a multimodality approach is often required.
- In cases involving chronic fistula tracts, de-epithelialization of the fistula tract before endoscopic closure can be achieved using argon plasma coagulation, an endoscopic brush, or with endoscopic resection of the fistula edges and/or fistula tract.

INTRODUCTION

Endoscopic suturing represents a highly versatile minimally invasive endoscopic surgical technique, with a wide range of applications throughout the gastrointestinal tract

Disclosures Statement: P.S. Ge has no conflicts of interest or financial ties to disclose. C.C. Thompson reports fees as a consultant from Boston Scientific and Medtronic; fees as a consultant and institutional grants from USGI Medical, Olympus America, and Apollo Endosurgery; and has a patent issued for Endoscopic Fistula Repair, held by Brigham and Women's Hospital.
[a] Department of Gastroenterology, Hepatology and Nutrition, The University of Texas MD Anderson Cancer Center, 1515 Holcombe Boulevard, Unit 1466, Houston, TX 77030-4009, USA;
[b] Division of Gastroenterology, Hepatology and Endoscopy, Brigham and Women's Hospital, 75 Francis Street, Boston, MA 02115, USA
* Corresponding author.
E-mail address: ccthompson@bwh.harvard.edu
twitter: @MetabolicEndo (C.C.T.)

Although several other platforms have been previously described, the Apollo Over-stitch and Overstitch SX (Apollo Endosurgery Inc, Austin, TX) are currently the only commercially available endoscopic suturing platforms. This article reviews the use of the Overstitch endoscopic suturing system specifically in the management of gastrointestinal perforations, leaks, and fistulas.

PERFORATIONS, LEAKS, AND FISTULAS

Gastrointestinal perforations are defined as an acute full-thickness defect of the gastrointestinal tract.[1] Perforation can occur as a result of a full-thickness injury, or progression from a partial thickness injury. Spontaneous perforations can result from a variety of etiologies including Boerhaave syndrome, ulcers, malignancy, diverticulitis, radiation therapy, inflammatory bowel disease, and intestinal ischemia. Traumatic perforations can result from direct blunt or penetrating trauma, or from foreign body ingestion. Accidental perforations are an uncommon but feared complication of endoscopic procedures, primarily those that are therapeutic in nature, such as in endoscopic dilation and resection. Etiologies of perforations are listed in **Box 1**.

Leaks are defined as a disruption in surgical anastomosis or closure, resulting in the egress and accumulation of luminal contents.[2] Leaks most often occur in an acute postoperative setting from gastrointestinal surgical procedures including intestinal resections and bariatric procedures. However, leaks can also occur from infection, inflammation, or diseases that increase intestinal pressure such as bowel obstruction. In a chronic setting, leaks can progress into fistulas, defined as the abnormal communication between 2 epithelialized surfaces. Chronic fistulas can involve communication with various different adjacent structures (eg, enteroenteric, enterobronchial/tracheal, enterovaginal, enterovesical, enterocutaneous, enteroatmospheric).

Perforations and leaks can present acutely, with sudden onset of chest or abdominal pain depending on the location of the perforation.[3] However, occasionally perforation can present in an indolent manner, presenting with sepsis, an abdominal mass, or fistula drainage. Fistulas will typically present with fevers, pain, and sequelae of fluid egress depending specifically on the location of the fistula (ie, diarrhea, cough, feculent vaginal or urinary discharge, cutaneous leakage).

APPROACH TO MANAGEMENT

The fundamental principles of perforation, leak, and fistula management include (1) identification of the site of disruption, (2) drainage of any leaked contents, and (3) controlling the flow of luminal contents with either diversion of luminal contents or closure of the disruption. Aside from management of the primary site of disruption, comprehensive management includes bowel rest, broad spectrum antibiotic therapy, fluid and electrolyte management, parenteral nutritional support, and drainage of any fluid collections and/or abscesses.[4,5]

When attempting endoscopic closure of an acute perforation, a sterile angiocatheter or Veress needle, connected to a syringe with sterile normal saline solution, can be placed into either the thoracic or peritoneal cavity through the chest or abdominal wall, to avoid complications associated with tension pneumothorax or tension pneumoperitoneum.

Traditionally, perforations, leaks, and fistulas require surgical management, especially if there is associated extraluminal contamination. However, the advent of endoscopic tools and techniques have allowed for select patients to be managed

---

Box 1
Etiologies of perforations

Spontaneous Perforation

Boerhaave syndrome (esophagus)

Diverticulitis

Inflammatory bowel disease

Intestinal ischemia

Malignancy

Perforated ulcer

Radiation therapy

Traumatic Perforation

Blunt trauma

Caustic injury

Foreign body ingestion

Penetrating trauma

Accidental Perforation

Endoscopy (EGD, colonoscopy, EUS, ERCP)

Endoscopic stricture management (dilation, bougienage, stricturotomy)

Endoscopic myotomy (POEM and related procedures)

Endoscopic resection (EMR, ESD, STER, EFTR)

Endoscopic treatment of gastrointestinal bleeding

Laparoscopic or open surgical injury

Other instrumentation (nasogastric tubes, Blakemore or Minnesota tubes, etc.)

Abbreviations: EFTR, endoscopic full-thickness resection; EGD, esophagogastroduodenoscopy; EMR, endoscopic mucosal resection; ERCP, endoscopic retrograde cholangiopancreatography; ESD, endoscopic submucosal dissection; EUS, endoscopic ultrasound; POEM, peroral endoscopic myotomy; STER, submucosal tunneling endoscopic resection.

---

endoscopically, with complex cases managed in a coordinated multidisciplinary effort involving surgery, interventional radiology, and endoscopy (**Box 2**).[6,7]

The decision between an endoscopic or surgical approach is dependent on the size and chronicity of the disruption, its location and endoscopic accessibility, and the ability to drain or limit any associated contamination. Endoscopic management can be a viable option for the management of acute perforations, with defect closure and/or diversion through enteral stent placement (**Box 3**). However, the management of leaks and fistulas are typically more complex and may require multimodality management in conjunction with interventional radiology and surgery.

ENDOSCOPIC SUTURING

Multiple endoscopic suturing devices have been described and developed over the past 2 decades, including the Bard EndoCinch (C.R. Bard, Murray Hill, NJ), the T-Bar (Cook Medical, Bloomington, IN), and the Eagle Claw (Olympus America, Center

---

Box 2
Approach to management of perforations, leaks, and fistulas

Clinical Management

Nothing by mouth

Fluid resuscitation

Intravenous broad spectrum antibiotics

Radiographic evaluation (plain films or contrast computed tomography scan)

Nasogastric decompression

Abdominal or chest decompression if tension pneumothorax or tension pneumoperitoneum

Intervention

Endoscopic therapy
   Immediate or early postprocedure recognition
   Contained or small/limited leak

Percutaneous or surgical intervention
   Delayed recognition
   Uncontained or large leak
   Clinical peritonitis

Box 3
Endoscopic tools and adjuncts for management of perforations, leaks, and fistulas

Diversion

Fully covered self-expanding metal stents

External Drainage

Percutaneous drainage (interventional radiology)

Surgical drainage

Internal Drainage

Endoscopic vacuum therapy

Transluminal pigtail plastic stents placed directly from lumen into fluid collections

De-Epithelialization (Fistulas)

Argon plasma coagulation of fistula edges

Endoscopic brushing of fistula tract

Endoscopic resection of fistula edges and/or fistula tract

Repair

Through the scope clips

Over the scope clips

Endoloop

Tissue sealants (eg, fibrin, cyanoacrylate)

Cardiac septal occluder

Endoscopic suturing (Overstitch)

Valley, PA) devices. The original devices were developed in support of natural orifice transluminal endoscopic surgery defect closures; however, each device had limitations that prevented further widespread use. The current Apollo Overstitch system was first developed in 2009, with a study from Moran and colleagues[8] demonstrating its use in placing full-thickness sutures for gastrotomy closure in a porcine model with satisfactory tissue apposition. Currently, the Overstitch is the only endoscopic suturing platform commercially available in the United States, with increasing applications such as in defect closure following endoscopic resection or peroral endoscopic myotomy (POEM), enteral stent fixation, and multiple bariatric endoscopy applications, in addition to the closure of perforations, leaks, and fistulas.[9]

The Overstitch system itself is a disposable single-use endoscopic suturing device (**Fig. 1**).[10] It is designed for use by a single operator, and allows full-thickness placement of either permanent (2–0 and 3–0 polypropylene) or absorbable (2–0 and 3–0 polydioxanone) sutures. The original Overstitch device requires a double-channel therapeutic endoscope. However, the newly introduced Overstitch SX device can be mounted alongside a single-channel endoscope and is compatible with more than 20 current single-channel flexible endoscopes and 4 platforms (Olympus, Pentax Medical, Fujifilm, and Storz) according to its manufacturer.

The main device is mounted on the tip of the double-channel therapeutic endoscope (Overstitch) or alongside a single-channel endoscope (Overstitch SX). The device contains a needle driver, which moves in an arclike fashion, and an anchor exchange catheter. The device is connected to a large handle, which is attached

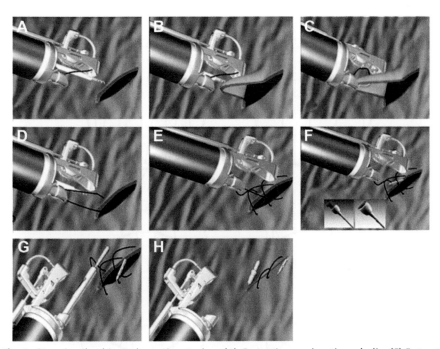

Fig. 1. Steps involved in endoscopic suturing. (*A*) Grasp tissue using tissue helix. (*B*) Retract tissue into the needle path. (*C*) Drive needle through the tissue. (*D*) Open needle arm to release tissue. (*E*) Repeat as indicated until suturing is complete. (*F*) Depress blue button to release needle. (*G*) Tighten and cinch. (*H*) Completed defect repair. (Courtesy of Apollo Endosurgery, Inc., Austin, TX; with permission.)

near the endoscope controls. The suture is first mounted onto the anchor exchange catheter and passed through the operating channel. The anchor is then transferred to the needle driver, and suturing is performed by transferring the anchor back and forth between the needle driver and the anchor exchange catheter. Tissue approximation can be facilitated with the use of a separate tissue helix, which is a corkscrewlike device that allows tissue grasping and retraction. When suturing is complete, a release button on the anchor exchange catheter releases the anchor. The suture is threaded onto a cinch device, which is then passed through the operating channel to both secure and cut the suture. In this fashion, the Overstitch device allows interrupted or continuous sutures to be placed without needing to remove the device (**Fig. 2**). The device itself can be reloaded multiple times with new needles without removing the endoscope.

ENDOSCOPIC SUTURING OF PERFORATIONS

Owing to the infrequency of iatrogenic perforations outside the setting of endoscopic mucosal resection (EMR) and endoscopic submucosal dissection (ESD) defect closure, and the relatively recent advent of endoscopic suturing, there is a paucity of literature evaluating the efficacy and outcomes of endoscopic suturing for perforations (**Fig. 3**), with existing literature confined to case studies, small case series, and animal studies. Indeed, in a Dutch systematic review of the existing literature published in 2015, which included 466 acute perforations across 24 different studies (21 retrospective, 3 prospective), perforations were closed using either standard

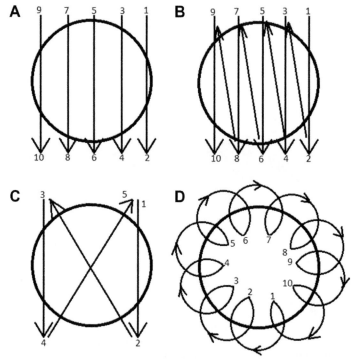

Fig. 2. Endoscopic suturing patterns. (*A*) Interrupted suture. (*B*) Running suture. (*C*) Figure-of-8 suture. (*D*) Pursestring suture.

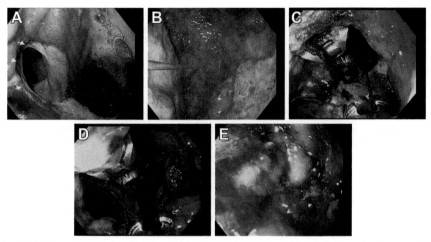

Fig. 3. Endoscopic sutured closure of a large perforation. (*A*) Initial view of a large perforated jejunal ulcer (arrows) within the proximal Roux limb in a patient with a history of Roux-en-Y gastric bypass surgery. (*B*) Endoscopic intraperitoneal exploration with washout and debridement of spilled luminal contents. (*C, D*) The perforation was closed using a single running suture. (*E*) Completed perforation closure.

endoclips, over the scope clips, or metal stents, and no cases involving endoscopic suturing were included.[11] As with the Dutch systematic review, most existing large series of endoscopic suturing for defect closure relate to closure of partial thickness defects due to EMR/ESD,[12] rather than acute full-thickness perforations.

The potential application of endoscopic suturing in the management of perforation was first described using previously available suturing platforms. Pham and colleagues[13] in 2006 described an animal study using the Eagle Claw prototype suturing device, considered to be the precursor of the currently available Overstitch device. In their study of 10 colonic perforations in 10 pigs, 8 perforations were successfully closed. Two perforations could not be closed due to device-related issues, resulting in worsening pneumoperitoneum and hemodynamic instability, and the animals were euthanized immediately. Of the 8 perforations that were closed, all of the pigs recovered well without any sepsis or peritonitis. On necropsy after 1 week, 7 out of 8 pigs had an intact perforation closure with no peritonitis or abscess formation; however, 1 pig demonstrated dehiscence of the perforation site. The results of the study demonstrated the feasibility of the prototype suturing device in closure of acute colonic perforations in a porcine model.

Other studies focused on competing endoscopic suturing-based tissue approximation systems. Sumiyama and colleagues[14] in 2007 described an animal study using a T-tag-based tissue approximation system. In their study of 12 gastric perforations in 6 pigs, all perforations were successfully closed and follow-up endoscopy and necropsy after 1 week demonstrated that the tissue anchors remained intact with firmly held sutures and sealed perforation. Raju and colleagues[15] in 2007 described an animal study comparing a similar full-thickness tissue approximation device versus a multi-clip applicator in closing 10 colon perforations. In their study, endoscopic closure of 4-cm-long colon perforations was successful in 9 out of 10 animals, with 1 failed closure using the multi-clip applicator. Successful closure prevented clinical peritonitis in 3 out of 4 animals in the suture closure group, and necropsy at 2 weeks showed mild peritonitis in 2 out of 4 animals; none developed fecal peritonitis.

Since the introduction of the Overstitch device, endoscopic suturing for perforations using the Overstitch device has mostly been limited to case studies or case series. In the esophagus, various groups have reported successful endoscopic suture repair of perforation during POEM for management of achalasia.[16,17] Henderson and colleagues[18] reported 3 cases of esophageal perforation in a 2014 case series, in which one patient had perforation due to Boerhaave syndrome, a second patient had perforation following unsuccessful endoscopic food disimpaction, and a third patient had perforation following transesophageal echocardiography. All 3 cases were successfully managed with endoscopic suturing with the Overstitch device. Maselli and colleagues[19] in 2017 reported 2 cases of successful endoscopic suture repair of esophageal perforations after failed attempts at surgical sutured closure. More recently, various groups have reported video case reports of successful suture repair of Boerhaave syndrome,[20] esophageal perforation from Savary dilation,[21] and type 1 duodenal perforation from duodenal stricture dilation.[22]

Occasionally, perforation closure may require diversion and/or management of leaked luminal contents. Diversion in the foregut can be accomplished with placement of a fully covered self-expanding metal stent, which can then be sutured in place to prevent migration.[23] Several groups have additionally reported direct abdominal exploration with washout of leaked luminal contents. Kumar and Thompson[24] reported 2 cases of perforation (1 gastric perforation and 1 gastrojejunal anastomotic perforation) in a 2014 case series, in which both cases were managed with endoscopic abdominal exploration through the perforation site to guide placement of an angiocatheter, inspect for any signs of injury that may warrant surgical management, and remove leaked luminal contents. Both perforations were then successfully repaired with endoscopic suturing with the Overstitch device, with confirmation of closure with an upper gastrointestinal (GI) series and discharge 1 day later. Moyer and colleagues[25] reported a recent series of 7 cases of endoscopic defect repair, which comprised of 4 perforations (1 esophageal perforation, 2 gastric perforations, and 1 duodenal perforation) and 3 postsurgical anastomotic leaks. In all cases, there was evidence of extraluminal contamination. The cases were then managed with transluminal washout, debridement, and either endoscopic sutured repair of the defect and/or endoscopic suturing of a fully covered self-expanding metal stent. Technical success was achieved in 100%, and overall clinical success in 86% due to 1 death from severe comorbid disease.

Several large retrospective case series have been published on endoscopic suturing for perforations. Kantsevoy and colleagues[26] in 2016 reported a series of 21 patients with iatrogenic colonic perforations from 2009 to 2014, of which 5 patients underwent closure with standard endoclips and 16 patients underwent closure with the Overstitch suturing device. The vast majority of the perforations were due to EMR/ESD; however, 2 were from screening colonoscopy and 1 was from colonic dilation. All 5 patients who underwent closure with endoclips subsequently had worsening abdominal pain. Four of those 5 patients required laparoscopy, which showed inadequate closure, thus requiring colon resection with ileocolonic anastomosis. One of those 5 patients underwent immediate rescue colonoscopy with endoscopic suturing, which was successful. On the other hand, only 2 patients who underwent closure with suturing subsequently had worsening abdominal pain, and laparoscopy confirmed complete and adequate closure. The results of the study demonstrated the apparent superiority of endoscopic suturing over standard endoclips for the management of colonic perforations, which are due to the ability of the Overstitch device to achieve full-thickness "surgical-quality" suturing and thus create an airtight closure. Stavropoulos and colleagues[9] in 2015 reported a large case series that included endoscopic suturing in 22 ESD defects, 24 endoscopic full-thickness resection defects, and 16 accidental perforations, all of which were successful with 2 minor adverse events. Similarly, Sharaiha and colleagues[23] in 2016 reported a multicenter case series on endoscopic suturing that included 47 cases for stent anchorage, 40 fistulas, 15 anastomotic leaks, and 20 perforations, and reported 93% clinical success in the management of perforations using endoscopic suturing.

Owing to publication bias, reported success rates of endoscopic suturing for repair of acute perforations are quite high. In an abstract from Bartell and colleagues[27] in 2018, which described a systematic review of patients who underwent endoscopic suturing for repair of acute perforations, the clinical success was reported to be greater than 98%. Although well-powered high quality studies are needed, prospective trials are unlikely to occur due to ethical issues of enrolling participants who are under sedation, unable to provide informed consent, and faced with a life-threatening adverse event that demands emergent attention.[28]

The optimal suturing approach for the closure of large perforations was studied in an ex vivo porcine model by Schulman and colleagues[29] in 2016. The study compared interrupted, running, horizontal mattress, and pursestring suturing patterns to close a 2-cm colon perforation, with subsequent measurement of mean pressure required to achieve air leakage. Their results demonstrated that a full-thickness running suture produced the most robust perforation closure, with highest leak pressure, and was completed in the shortest amount of time.

ENDOSCOPIC SUTURING OF LEAKS AND FISTULAS

Endoscopic suturing has been used in the management of leaks and fistulas, both in the acute and chronic setting (**Fig. 4**), with variable success. As with the endoscopic

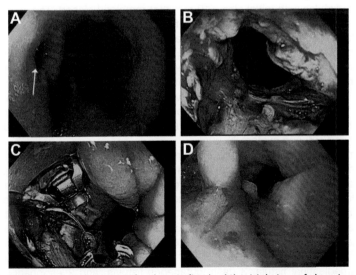

Fig. 4. Endoscopic sutured closure of a chronic fistula. (*A*) Initial view of chronic gastrogastric fistula (arrow) in a patient with a history of Roux-en-Y gastric bypass surgery. (*B*) An endoscopic fistulectomy is performed using a modified ESD technique to de-epithelialize the fistula tract. (*C*) The fistula was closed using 2 sets of running sutures in a layered fashion. (*D*) Completed fistula closure.

management of perforations, there is an overall paucity of literature evaluating the efficacy and outcomes of endoscopic suturing for leaks and fistulas, with existing literature confined to case studies, small case series, and animal studies. Given the challenging nature of endoscopic therapy for leaks and fistulas, endoscopic suturing is typically a component of a carefully selected multimodality approach that may also include argon plasma coagulation (APC), through the scope clips, over the scope clips, and glue.[30] Diversion of enteral contents with placement of a fully covered self-expanding metal stent (which can then be sutured in place to prevent migration) is often a necessary adjunct.[23] In addition, percutaneous drainage catheters placed by interventional radiology or surgery are commonly necessary to evacuate cavities and fluid collections.[5] Although successful closure using endoscopic suturing has been described in the literature, fistula/leak recurrence may develop and additional therapy may be required, particularly among challenging chronic epithelialized fistulas, which may be exceptionally resistant to closure.

The overall experience with endoscopic suturing for fistula closure varies by the type of fistula involved. Gastrogastric fistulas, a known complication from Roux-en-Y gastric bypass, has thus far been the most commonly reported scenario for endoscopic sutured fistula closure. Spaun and colleagues[31] in 2010 reported closure for 4 patients with 5 gastrogastric fistulas using the T-tag–based tissue apposition system. Although primary closure of the 5 fistulas was 100%, after 3 months only the smallest fistula (10 mm) remained closed, and after 6 months all fistulas had reopened, leading the investigators to conclude that permanent closure could not be achieved. In a much larger series, Fernandez-Esparrach and colleagues[32] in 2010 reported closure for 95 patients with gastrogastric fistulas using either standard clips (24/95, 25%) or the Bard EndoCinch suturing system (71/95, 75%). Complete initial fistula closure was achieved in 95% of patients; however, 65% of fistulas reopened in an average of 177 days. In an average follow-up period of 395 days, it was noted that none of the fistulas with initial size greater than 20 mm remained closed, compared with 32% of the fistulas with initial size ≤10 mm that remained closed. The investigators therefore concluded that the best results for endoscopic fistula closure were seen with fistulas ≤10 mm in diameter. More recently, Wu and colleagues[33] in 2016 reported a patient with a 2-cm gastrogastric fistula that was successfully closed with the Overstitch suturing device, using a single polydiaxonone suture in a figure-of-8 configuration, and that remained closed on 6-month follow-up. Additional abstracts have also reported successful use of the Overstitch suturing device in closure of gastrogastric fistulas,[34] including a matched-cohort study, which demonstrated the superiority of the full-thickness Overstitch suturing device compared with a superficial suction-based suturing system.[35]

Aside from gastrogastric fistulas, closures of various other enteric fistulas have been reported using the Overstitch system. Kantsevoy and Thuluvath[36] reported a chronic gastrocutaneous fistula from prior gastrostomy tube that had been resistant to prior closure attempts with clips and glue. The fistula was successfully closed using 3 separate sutures deployed using the Overstitch system, without further drainage at 1-month follow-up. Several other case reports have described successful gastrocutaneous fistula closure using the Overstitch device.[37,38] Catalano and colleagues[39] reported successful closure of 6 various enteric fistulas, including an esophagomediastinal fistula, 3 gastrocutaneous fistulas, and 2 esophagobronchial fistulas; the esophagobronchial fistulas notably required 3 to 4 sessions for complete closure. Stavropoulos and colleagues[9] reported successful closure of 2 leaks and 12 fistulas (9 from gastric sleeves, 2 from Roux-en-Y gastric bypass, and 1 post-gastrostomy tube removal), and demonstrated 100% closure among the 2 leaks and 83% closure among the 12 fistulas. In the multicenter case series reported by Sharaiha and colleagues,[23] among 40 fistulas and 15 anastomotic leaks, the clinical success rate was 80% and 27%, respectively.

Additional case reports have described the use of the Overstitch device to successfully close a persistent esophagopleural fistula from Boerhaave syndrome,[40] a gastropleural fistula from a deformed sleeve gastrectomy,[41] a cholecystoduodenal fistula,[42] a gastropulmonary fistula following esophagectomy,[43] and a malignant gastroretroperitoneal fistula from primary gastric lymphoma.[44]

In cases in which the fistula tract has epithelialized, it is important to attempt to de-epithelialize the fistula tract before endoscopic closure. De-epithelialization is traditionally achieved using either APC along the perimeter of the fistula, or mechanical abrasion of the fistula tract and perimeter using a brush. Abidi and Thompson[45] in 2016 described a novel technique involving a modified ESD technique to fully resect a gastrogastric fistula tract, followed by sutured closure using the Overstitch device. Pang and colleagues[46] in 2018 described a similar technique in the closure of a chronic tracheoesophageal fistula, which involved multiple small snare mucosal resections around the fistula opening on the esophageal side, followed by successful sutured closure using the Overstitch device.

The largest existing multicenter series describing the use of endoscopic suturing in the management of gastrointestinal fistulas was reported by Mukewar and colleagues[47] in 2016. The series included 56 patients from 3 hospitals, and comprised a wide variety of gastrointestinal fistulas, including gastrogastric fistulas, enteroperitoneal fistulas, enterovaginal fistulas, enterobronchial fistulas, enterocutaneous fistulas, and leaks. Gastrogastric fistulas were the most common etiology (51.8%), and 28.6% patients had undergone prior failed attempts at closure. Although immediate success was achieved using endoscopic suturing in all patients (100%), durable closure was observed in only 22.4% at 12 months, with a 17.1% ongoing closure rate of gastrogastric fistulas and 31.4% closure rate of other fistulas. Of the original 56 patients, 13 patients (30.2%) were able to achieve closure without the need for additional therapies, whereas 17 patients required additional attempts, of which successful closure was attained in only 4 out of 17 patients. The remaining patients either were lost to follow-up or had unsuccessful attempts at fistula closure. One patient with an enteroperitoneal fistula underwent 5 attempts at fistula closure, all of which were ultimately unsuccessful. Although the study overall demonstrates the feasibility of endoscopic suturing for fistula closure, the relatively low rate of durable closure highlights the fundamental challenges of fistula closure.

Although Overstitch has been well described for fistulas, endoscopic suturing can also be applied to acute leaks and dehiscence. Belfiori and colleagues[48] in 2017 described using the Overstitch device to close a large anastomotic dehiscence 1 week following left colectomy for colon cancer. The perimeter of the leak was first cauterized with APC, and subsequently running sutures were placed using the Overstitch device in a distal-to-proximal technique, attempting to create a full-thickness suture repair. A minimal residual leak was noted 1 week later, and a second round of endoscopic sutured repair was performed with the Overstitch device. This ultimately resulted in a successful and durable closure at 6-month follow-up. Although successful, it is important to note that an abdominal surgical drain had remained in place for removal of soiled contents that had leaked into the peritoneum.

Irrespective of the method of endoscopic closure for fistulas and leaks, successful closure of fistulas and leaks requires adequate drainage of any leaked luminal contents. This is typically achieved using either surgical drainage or percutaneous drainage placed by an interventional radiologist. However, recently internal drainage techniques have also been described using either endoscopic stents placed into adjacent fluid collections,[49,50] or endoscopic vacuum therapy.[51,52]

LIMITATIONS

Despite the advantages and robustness of endoscopic suturing, there remain multiple limitations to the Overstitch device. The current Overstitch device is limited to the Olympus double-channel therapeutic endoscope, whereas the Overstitch SX device is compatible with multiple platforms of single-channel endoscopes. However, neither device is compatible with colonoscopes. Both devices are characterized by their large size and limited field of view, and the Overstitch SX device appears to have an even more limited maneuverability when compared with the original Overstitch device due to its design. Because of these issues, the ability to suture defects and perforations in certain challenging locations remains limited to all but the most experienced operators. Difficult locations for endoscopic suturing includes the gastric fundus (because of poor angulation/maneuverability), duodenum (because of narrow space), and the right colon (because of incompatibility with colonoscopes).

In addition, despite its availability, the Overstitch device demands familiarity with the device for optimal results, especially with regard to the ability to place full-thickness sutures and the ability to perform complex suturing patterns. Although different situations may require different approaches, endoscopic suturing for perforations is typically best performed in a right-to-left and distal-to-proximal progression, using a running suture pattern.[29] This allows a robust closure and also maintains clear visibility of the defect edges until the suturing has been completed. On the other hand, due to the circular shape of the defect, endoscopic suturing for fistulas may be best performed in a figure-of-8 pattern. This allows equal circumferential anisotropic compression from the suture toward the center of the defect.[9] However, either of these complex suturing patterns can be prone to entanglement of the suture especially in the hands of an inexperienced operator, and any suture failure via tissue erosion or suture breakage would result in dehiscence of the entire closure. Similarly, accidental needle drop or breakage of the suture during cinching could result in failure of the entire closure.

SUMMARY

Endoscopic suturing represents an important technological advancement in the minimally invasive management of perforations, fistulas, and leaks. The currently available Overstitch platform is more complex than traditional through the scope and over the scope clips deployment, and requires additional training and experience to achieve proficiency. Despite this, with familiarity and mastery of the device, Overstitch allows for the capability to mimic a true full-thickness surgical closure in a minimally invasive endoscopic fashion. Although the present data suggest that endoscopic suturing is favorable in the management of perforations, it remains challenging and suboptimal in the long-term management of chronic fistulas. Further prospective comparative studies are needed to define the role of endoscopic suturing and determine its long-term outcomes in the management of perforations, fistulas, and leaks.

REFERENCES

1. Bemelman WA, Baron TH. Endoscopic management of transmural defects, including leaks, perforations, and fistulae. Gastroenterology 2018;154(7): 1938–46.e1.

2. Goenka MK, Goenka U. Endotherapy of leaks and fistula. World J Gastrointest Endosc 2015;7(7):702–13.
3. Baron TH, Wong Kee Song LM, Zielinski MD, et al. A comprehensive approach to the management of acute endoscopic perforations (with videos). Gastrointest Endosc 2012;76(4):838–59.
4. Rogalski P, Daniluk J, Baniukiewicz A, et al. Endoscopic management of gastrointestinal perforations, leaks and fistulas. World J Gastroenterol 2015;21(37): 10542.
5. Muniraj T, Aslanian HR. The use of OverStitchTM for the treatment of intestinal perforation, fistulas and leaks. Gastrointest Interv 2017;6(3):151–6.
6. Stavropoulos SN, Modayil R, Friedel D. Closing perforations and postperforation management in endoscopy: esophagus and stomach. Gastrointest Endosc Clin N Am 2015;25(1):29–45.
7. Boumitri C, Kumta NA, Patel M, et al. Closing perforations and postperforation management in endoscopy: duodenal, biliary, and colorectal. Gastrointest Endosc Clin N Am 2015;25(1):47–54.
8. Moran EA, Gostout CJ, Bingener J. Preliminary performance of a flexible cap and catheter-based endoscopic suturing system. Gastrointest Endosc 2009;69(7): 1375–83.
9. Stavropoulos SN, Modayil R, Friedel D. Current applications of endoscopic suturing. World J Gastrointest Endosc 2015;7(8):777.
10. ASGE Technology Committee, Banerjee S, Barth BA, Bhat YM, et al. Endoscopic closure devices. Gastrointest Endosc 2012;76(2):244–51.
11. Verlaan T, Voermans RP, van Berge Henegouwen MI, et al. Endoscopic closure of acute perforations of the GI tract: a systematic review of the literature. Gastrointest Endosc 2015;82(4):618–28.e5.
12. Kantsevoy SV, Bitner M, Mitrakov AA, et al. Endoscopic suturing closure of large mucosal defects after endoscopic submucosal dissection is technically feasible, fast, and eliminates the need for hospitalization (with videos). Gastrointest Endosc 2014;79(3):503–7.
13. Pham BV, Raju GS, Ahmed I, et al. Immediate endoscopic closure of colon perforation by using a prototype endoscopic suturing device: feasibility and outcome in a porcine model (with video). Gastrointest Endosc 2006;64(1):113–9.
14. Sumiyama K, Gostout CJ, Rajan E, et al. Endoscopic full-thickness closure of large gastric perforations by use of tissue anchors. Gastrointest Endosc 2007; 65(1):134–9.
15. Raju GS, Shibukawa G, Ahmed I, et al. Endoluminal suturing may overcome the limitations of clip closure of a gaping wide colon perforation (with videos). Gastrointest Endosc 2007;65(6):906–11.
16. Kurian AA, Bhayani NH, Reavis K, et al. Endoscopic suture repair of full-thickness esophagotomy during per-oral esophageal myotomy for achalasia. Surg Endosc 2013;27(10):3910.
17. Modayil R, Friedel D, Stavropoulos SN. Endoscopic suture repair of a large mucosal perforation during peroral endoscopic myotomy for treatment of achalasia. Gastrointest Endosc 2014;80(6):1169–70.
18. Henderson JB, Sorser SA, Atia AN, et al. Repair of esophageal perforations using a novel endoscopic suturing system. Gastrointest Endosc 2014;80(3):535.
19. Maselli R, Viale E, Fanti L, et al. Successful endoscopic suturing of esophageal perforation after surgical suturing failure. Endoscopy 2017;49(09):E202–3.
20. Chen A, Kim R. Boerhaave syndrome treated with endoscopic suturing. VideoGIE 2019;4(3):118–9.

21. Avila N, Schwartz A, Tarnasky P, et al. Urgent esophageal repair with endoscopic suturing. VideoGIE 2018;3(3):77–8.
22. Hyun JJ, Kozarek RA, Irani SS. Endoscopic suturing of a large type I duodenal perforation. VideoGIE 2019;4(2):78–80.
23. Sharaiha RZ, Kumta NA, DeFilippis EM, et al. A large multicenter experience with endoscopic suturing for management of gastrointestinal defects and stent anchorage in 122 patients: a retrospective review. J Clin Gastroenterol 2016; 50(5):388–92.
24. Kumar N, Thompson CC. A novel method for endoscopic perforation management by using abdominal exploration and full-thickness sutured closure. Gastrointest Endosc 2014;80(1):156–61.
25. Moyer MT, Chintanaboina J, Walsh LT, et al. Transluminal washout and debridement of extraluminal contamination as an adjunct to endoscopic defect repair. VideoGIE 2019;4(2):91–4.
26. Kantsevoy SV, Bitner M, Hajiyeva G, et al. Endoscopic management of colonic perforations: clips versus suturing closure (with videos). Gastrointest Endosc 2016;84(3):487–93.
27. Bartell N, Kaul V, Kothari TH, et al. Gastrointestinal perforation closure using over-the-scope clips and endoscopic suturing: a systematic review. Gastrointest Endosc 2018;87(6):AB248–9.
28. Stavropoulos SN, Friedel D. Closing acute iatrogenic perforations: there are holes in the data! Gastrointest Endosc 2015;82(4):629–30.
29. Schulman A, Aihara H, Chiang AL, et al. Endoscopic suturing for large colonic perforations. Gastrointest Endosc 2016;83(5):AB503.
30. Willingham FF, Buscaglia JM. Endoscopic management of gastrointestinal leaks and fistulae. Clin Gastroenterol Hepatol 2015;13(10):1714–21.
31. Spaun GO, Martinec DV, Kennedy TJ, et al. Endoscopic closure of gastrogastric fistulas by using a tissue apposition system (with videos). Gastrointest Endosc 2010;71(3):606–11.
32. Fernandez-Esparrach G, Lautz DB, Thompson CC. Endoscopic repair of gastrogastric fistula after Roux-en-Y gastric bypass: a less-invasive approach. Surg Obes Relat Dis 2010;6(3):282–8.
33. Wu E, Garberoglio R, Scharf K. Endoluminal closure of gastrogastric fistula. Surg Obes Relat Dis 2016;12(3):705–6.
34. Watson RR, Jirapinyo P, Thompson CC. Endoscopic repair of post-operative gastrointestinal fistulae using a novel endoscopic suturing device: technical feasibility and safety. Gastroenterology 2011;140(5):S—118.
35. Tuyama AC, Kumar N, Aihara H, et al. Endoscopic repair of gastrogastric fistula after roux-en-Y gastric bypass: a matched cohort study evaluating two methods of fistula closure. Gastroenterology 2013;144(5):S—220.
36. Kantsevoy SV, Thuluvath PJ. Successful closure of a chronic refractory gastrocutaneous fistula with a new endoscopic suturing device (with video). Gastrointest Endosc 2012;75(3):688–90.
37. Armengol-Miro JR, Dot J, Abu-Suboh Abadia M, et al. New endoscopic suturing device for closure of chronic gastrocutaneous fistula in an immunocompromised patient. Endoscopy 2011;43(Suppl 2 UCTN):E403–4.
38. Stanich PP, Sklaw B, Krishna SG. Persistent peristomal leakage from percutaneous endoscopic gastrostomy successfully treated with endoscopic suturing. Endoscopy 2013;45(Suppl 2 UCTN):E394.

39. Catalano MF, Sorser SA, Henderson JB, et al. Successful closure of enteric fistulas using the Apollo Overstitch Suturing System. Gastroenterology 2014; 146(5). S-142–3.
40. Bonin EA, Wong Kee Song LM, Gostout ZS, et al. Closure of a persistent esophagopleural fistula assisted by a novel endoscopic suturing system. Endoscopy 2012;44(Suppl 2 UCTN):E8–9.
41. Andrawes S, El Douaihy Y. Using the endoscopic overstitching device and fully covered esophageal stents for closure of a gastropleural fistula and repair of a deformed gastric sleeve. VideoGIE 2017;2(5):98–9.
42. Shah-Khan S, Vallabh H, Cardinal J, et al. Novel use of an endoscopic suturing device to repair a Cholecystoduodenal Fistula. ACG Case Rep J 2017;4:e121.
43. Chon SH, Toex U, Plum PS, et al. Successful closure of a gastropulmonary fistula after esophagectomy using the Apollo Overstitch and endoscopic vacuum therapy. Endoscopy 2018;50(7):E149–50.
44. Alshati A, Sachdev MS, Tan A, et al. Successful endoscopic management of a malignant gastroretroperitoneal fistula. VideoGIE 2019;4(3):123–5.
45. Abidi WM, Thompson CC. Endoscopic treatment of a chronic fistula by resection and sutured closure. Gastrointest Endosc 2016;83(5):1031–2.
46. Pang M, Mousa O, Werlang M, et al. A hybrid endoscopic technique to close tracheoesophageal fistula. VideoGIE 2018;3(1):15–6.
47. Mukewar S, Kumar N, Catalano M, et al. Safety and efficacy of fistula closure by endoscopic suturing: a multi-center study. Endoscopy 2016;48(11):1023–8.
48. Belfiori V, Antonini F, Deminicis S, et al. Successful closure of anastomotic dehiscence after colon-rectal cancer resection using the Apollo overstitch suturing system. Endoscopy 2017;49(8):823–4.
49. de Moura DT, Sachdev AH, Thompson CC. Endoscopic full-thickness defects and closure techniques. Curr Treat Options Gastroenterol 2018;16(4):386–405.
50. Gonzalez JM, Lorenzo D, Guilbaud T, et al. Internal endoscopic drainage as first line or second line treatment in case of postsleeve gastrectomy fistulas. Endosc Int Open 2018;6(6):E745–50.
51. Kuehn F, Janisch F, Schwandner F, et al. Endoscopic vacuum therapy in colorectal surgery. J Gastrointest Surg 2016;20(2):328–34.
52. Kuehn F, Loske G, Schiffmann L, et al. Endoscopic vacuum therapy for various defects of the upper gastrointestinal tract. Surg Endosc 2017;31(9):3449–58.

The Use of the Overstitch to Close Endoscopic Resection Defects

Jennifer M. Kolb, MD, Hazem Hammad, MD*

KEYWORDS

- Endoscopic mucosal resection • Endoscopic submucosal dissection
- Resection defect • Endoscopic clip • Endoscopic suturing

KEY POINTS

- Endoscopic mucosal resection and endoscopic submucosal dissection are safe and effective techniques for removal of gastrointestinal neoplasia.
- The most common adverse events include bleeding and perforation, which can be immediate or delayed. Use of conventional endoclips or modified approaches using endoloop and clips can decrease this risk.
- The Overstitch (Apollo Endosurgery, Austin, TX) endoscopic suturing device offers a novel approach for closure of the resection defect. Although limited data are available, initial experience with this technique demonstrates safety and high efficacy.
- Our approach is to start with the edge most distal to the scope insertion site (antegrade position). Sutures are placed through the mucosal and submucosal flat at the edge of the resection, as opposed to the muscle layer.
- We mostly use a single stitch in a continuous running fashion avoiding significant narrowing of the lumen.

 Video content accompanies this article at http://www.giendo.theclinics.com.

INTRODUCTION

Endoscopic resection of luminal gastrointestinal neoplasia offers a minimally invasive, lower risk alternative to surgery that can be highly successful in the appropriate setting. The concept and techniques were pioneered by our colleagues in Asia in

Disclosure Statement: J.M. Kolb is supported in part by the NIH Gastrointestinal Diseases Training Grant (T32-DK007038). H. Hammad is a consultant for Olympus, Wilson Cook and Medtronics.
Division of Gastroenterology and Hepatology, University of Colorado Hospital, Anschutz Medical Campus, 1635 Aurora Court, F735, Aurora, CO 80045, USA
* Corresponding author.
E-mail address: hazem.hammad@ucdenver.edu

the 1990s and have since gained momentum in the United States as an organ-sparing, first-line approach for many clinical scenarios, including Barrett's esophagus-related neoplasia, superficial squamous cell carcinoma of the esophagus, early gastric adenocarcinoma, duodenal adenomas, and colorectal neoplasia.

Advanced endoscopic resection draws on a long history of standard polypectomy performed during routine colonoscopy. Recognition of flat or sessile polyps prompted development of a new technique called endoscopic mucosal resection (EMR), which uses special tools to lift up the lesion and limit damage to the underlying gastrointestinal wall. EMR techniques include injection-assisted EMR, cap-assisted EMR, ligation-assisted EMR, and underwater EMR.[1] Endoscopic resection techniques also include endoscopic submucosal dissection (ESD). ESD has the added advantage over EMR that larger, histologically more advanced lesions can be resected en bloc, preserving the lateral resection margins for histologic assessment. This procedure provides more confidence in the diagnosis of a T1 lesion and ensures complete removal with subsequent significantly lower rates of neoplasia recurrence. ESD can potentially achieve a complete (R0) oncologic resection with curative intent.

ADVERSE EVENTS OF ENDOSCOPIC MUCOSAL RESECTION AND ENDOSCOPIC SUBMUCOSAL DISSECTION

The most common adverse events that occur with EMR and ESD include bleeding, perforation, and stricture formation. Intraprocedural bleeding or perforation can generally be treated endoscopically, whereas delayed presentations might require additional therapies.

Bleeding

Bleeding is the most common adverse event associated with endoscopic resection. EMR related bleeding occurs most commonly in the duodenum (11.5%–19.3% for lesions <3 cm) followed by the colon and stomach (approximately 11%), and rarely in the esophagus (1.2%).[2] The rates of intraprocedural and delayed bleeding with EMR of large colorectal lesions ranges from 1% to 11%, but there is a wide variation with some studies suggesting higher risk.[3,4] Predictors for immediate bleeding include polyp morphology (Paris classification 0-IIa + Is; odds ratio [OR], 2.12; $P = .004$), villous histology (OR, 1.84; $P = .007$), large lesions (OR, 1.24/10 mm; $P<.001$), proximal location, and lower volume centers.[5,6] Intraprocedural bleeding and proximal colon location (OR, 3.72; $P<.001$) are risk factors for postprocedural bleeding.[5] A similar trend was seen in a large study of 477 patients who underwent gastric EMR where delayed bleeding occurred in 5.3% of patients and the strongest predictor was the presence of immediate bleeding.[7] EMR for nonampullary duodenal polyps is particularly high risk for bleeding, especially in lesions measuring greater than 3 cm.[8]

Intraprocedural bleeding during ESD is generally expected and can be managed with coagulation through the ESD knife or coagulation forceps. Delayed bleeding after ESD occurs most commonly with gastric lesions (4.5%–15.6%)[9] compared with colorectal (2%) or esophageal sites (0%–5.3%).[10,11] Antacid therapy can be used to decrease the risk of post-ESD gastric ulcer formation.[12] In a large study of ESD for 377 colorectal lesions, delayed bleeding occurred at a rate of 6.6% and was associated with rectal location and submucosal fibrosis.[13]

Perforation

Perforation rates with colon EMR are low, but early identification is critical. Careful examination of the postresection site in the colon (or on the resected specimen) can identify a classic target sign suggesting resection through the muscular propria[14] **(Fig. 1)**. Prompt recognition and placement of conventional endoscopic clips is generally adequate to seal a small defect in the muscle layer. A meta-analysis examining outcomes in colorectal ESD showed pooled perforation rates of 4%.[10]

Perforation is uncommon with gastric EMR (<1%), but pooled risk in meta-analyses point to 4.5 times higher rates with gastric ESD.[9,15] Gastric perforations of less than 1 cm can be successfully managed with endoscopic clips the majority of the time and an omental patch can be helpful for larger perforations.[16] Perforation with esophageal EMR is rare but nearly 2-fold higher with esophageal ESD (pooled perforation rate of 2.3%).[11,17]

TECHNIQUES TO DECREASE ADVERSE EVENTS
Prophylactic Clipping

The relatively high rates of bleeding associated with EMR of large colorectal lesions prompted multiple observational studies evaluating the use of prophylactic clipping. In 2015, Zhang and colleagues[18] performed the first prospective, randomized controlled study comparing clip closure of resection defects (EMR and ESD) compared with no closure in 348 patients with large (1–4 cm) colorectal tumors. The rate of delayed bleeding was significantly lower in the clip compared with no clip group (1.1% vs 6.9%; $P = .01$). Subjects in the clip group also had shorter hospital stay (3.1 vs 4.7 days; $P = .03$), less abdominal pain (2.8% vs 16.7%; $P<.01$), and higher patient satisfaction. Results from a recent multicenter randomized clinical trial of clip closure versus no closure for large ($\geq$20 mm) nonpedunculated colorectal polyps demonstrated lower rates of postprocedure bleeding with clip closure (3.5% vs 7.1%; absolute risk difference, 3.6%; 95% confidence interval, 0.7%–6.5%) independent of antithrombotic medications or polyp size.[19] The impact of clipping seems to be driven largely by benefit for proximal polyps (3.3% vs 9.6%; absolute risk difference, 6.3%; 95% confidence interval, 2.5%–10.1%).

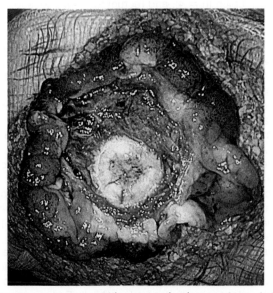

Fig. 1. A classic "target sign" seen on the resected colon specimen, indicating resection through and defect in the muscularis propria (perforation).

Modified Techniques for Larger Defects

Conventional endoclips can typically achieve successful closure of defects up to 2 cm; however, adaptations to the design allow for closure of even larger mucosal defects. In 2004, Matsuda and colleagues[20] demonstrated a new technique using the endoloop and clips using a double channel endoscope to close a large 5 cm mucosal defect after colonic EMR.

Adaptations to the endoloop system enabled closure through a single channel colonoscope. The predetached endoloop strategy was used to close right sided colonic ESD defects in 18 patients without any immediate or delayed complications.[21] A similar method has also been used to successfully close gastric perforations with no delayed complications even in patients on anticoagulation.[22,23] Data for use of other successful technologies[24] including over the scope clips for closing ESD defects[25,26] is presented in an earlier chapter.

Endoscopic Suturing to Close Resection Defects

The Overstitch (Apollo Endosurgery, Austin, TX) endoscopic suturing device is the only currently available device approved by the US Food and Drug Administration to close perforations, fistulas, and for bariatric endoscopy. An overview of its development and applications is described in previous chapters. Herein we focus on its potential to close endoscopic resection defects.

As compared with endoscopic clips or endoloops that were designed for hemostasis, endoscopic suturing is intended for tissue apposition and thus can effectively close a large defect. Although currently not standard of care for closure of ESD defects, this technique has potential—in the hands of expert endoscopists—to decrease adverse events and reduce or eliminate hospitalization, thereby reducing costs.[27,28]

Limited data are available on the efficacy of endoscopic suturing after ESD and no standard technique currently exists for this indication. In a retrospective single-center study by Kantsevoy and colleagues,[29] 12 patients underwent ESD of 3–8 cm lesions in the stomach (n = 4), colon (n = 4), and rectum (n = 4). Endoscopic suturing of the post-ESD defect was performed with use of a double channel endoscope and the Overstitch system with either a continuous suture line or separated stitches. The technical success rate was 100% and accomplished efficiently with a mean closure time of 10.0 ± 5.8 minutes per patient. The average cost of closure using 1 suture and cinch approximated $875 per patient (equivalent cost to 5–6 endoclips), but afforded greater cost savings by allowing all patients to be discharged on the same day. None of the patients experienced any immediate or delayed adverse events, including bleeding or perforation. In a retrospective analysis comparing clipping versus suturing to close iatrogenic colonic perforations in 21 patients (11 related to ESD and 5 related to EMR), primary closure was performed with endoscopic clips in 5 patients and endoscopic suturing in 16 patients. All patients who underwent clip closure had worsening abdominal pain after the procedure, 4 patients required laparoscopy and 1 patient required rescue colonoscopy with endoscopic suturing. In the suturing group, 2 patients had abdominal pain after the procedure and underwent diagnostic laparoscopy, which confirmed adequate complete endoscopic closure. The other 14 patients did not require any further intervention.[30]

The steps for using the Overstitch device have been previously described.[31] In our institution, upon completion of the ESD procedure in either the stomach or rectum, we use the double-channel therapeutic gastroscope (Olympus, Tokyo, Japan) loaded with the OverStitch endoscopic suturing system (Apollo Endosurgery). Suturing is typically performed in the antegrade position. Starting with the edge most distal to the

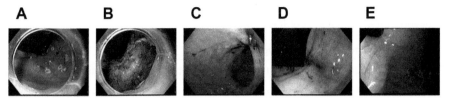

Fig. 2. (*A*) Marking of a Paris IIa nodule at the incisura/proximal gastric antrum. Biopsies showed carcinoma. (*B*) Post-ESD defect. (*C*) ESD defect after suturing, forward view. (*D*) ESD defect after suturing, retroflex view. (*E*) Follow-up endoscopy 6 months later demonstrates a well-healed scar at the resection site.

scope insertion site, endoscopic suturing of the ESD defect is initiated. The suture is typically placed through the mucosal and submucosal flap at the edge of the resection, as opposed to the muscle layer (Videos 1 and 2). This technique of suturing is used to maintain visualization throughout the entire suturing process, facilitate handling of the endoscope with the suturing system and avoid significant narrowing of the lumen at the end of the suturing. As shown in the video, we typically use a single stitch in a continuous running suture line moving side to side down the resection defect and eventually secure the suture with 1 cinch.

Similar suturing technique can be applied after gastric (**Fig. 2**), duodenal (**Fig. 3**), and colon resection procedures (EMR and ESD). Healing of mucosal defects after

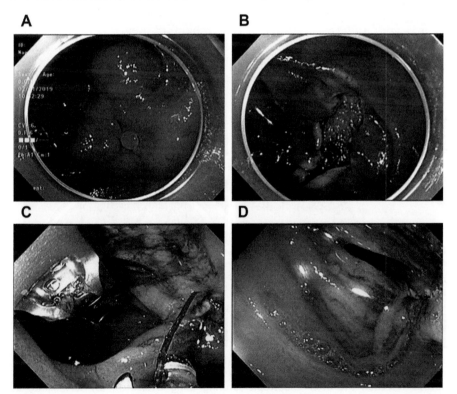

Fig. 3. Suturing after duodenal EMR. (*A*) A 3-cm sessile polypoid lesion in the second portion of the duodenum. (*B*) Resection defect after EMR. (*C*) Suturing of EMR defect. (*D*) Resection site after defect closure with suturing. ([*C*] *Courtesy of* Apollo Endosurgery, Inc., Austin, TX.)

endoscopic suturing does not seem to affect endoscopic surveillance, visualization, or sampling of the resection scar (**Fig. 4**).

Advantages to Endoscopic Suturing

Endoscopic closure of large resection defects can be useful for multiple reasons:

1. Most patients can be discharged the same day.
2. Suturing could potentially decrease the risk of adverse events. This is particularly helpful in elderly patients with comorbidities where severe adverse events such as major bleeding or perforation could be life threatening.

Our initial experience and observation with this technique (14 patients) allowed a large number of patients to be discharged the same day without the need for inpatient observation.[32]

Limitations of Endoscopic Suturing

As mentioned, the currently available Overstitch device is only used with a gastro-scope; therefore, suturing in the proximal colon could be limited if the gastroscope

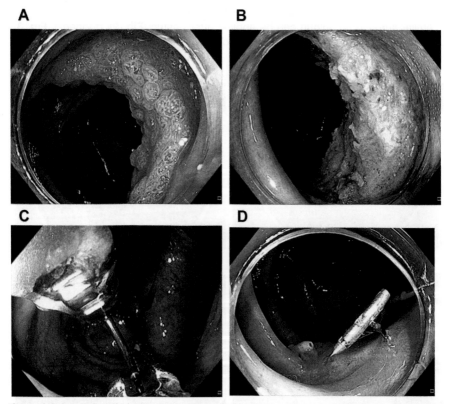

Fig. 4. (*A*) A 5-cm sessile lesion at the hepatic flexure in a 41-year-old patient with Crohn's colitis. Biopsies showed low-grade dysplasia. (*B*) Wide-field mucosal resection site. (*C*) Mucosal resection site after endoscopic suturing using Overstitch. (*D*) Surveillance at 6 months showed a well-healed EMR scar with sutures in place. The sutures were removed and evaluation of the scar (endoscopic and histopathologic) showed no residual dysplasia. ([*C, D*] *Courtesy of* Apollo Endosurgery, Inc., Austin, TX.)

cannot be inserted to that area. The use of an overtube system such as DiLumen (Lumendi, Westport, CT) could make insertion of the overstitch device to the right colon easier.

The use of Overstitch to close endoscopic resection defects prolongs the duration (need to switch scopes and the duration of suturing) and increases the cost of the procedure. Suturing after endoscopic resection typically takes around 10 minutes. The cost effectiveness of suturing all endoscopic resection defects (vs high-risk patients) needs to be further evaluated.

Although we have not seen any adverse events from endoscopic suturing of resection defects, adverse events could potentially include pain, bleeding, perforation, infection/sepsis, and injury to nearby intra-abdominal organs.

The Overstitch device requires special training and should be performed by an experienced endoscopist who is proficient in endoscopic suturing. Endoscopic suturing is technically challenging but can be learned through observation of experienced endoscopists and hands-on experience on ex vivo models.

SUPPLEMENTARY DATA

Supplementary data related to this article can be found online at https://doi.org/10.1016/j.giec.2019.08.006.

REFERENCES

1. Binmoeller KF, Weilert F, Shah J, et al. Underwater" EMR without submucosal injection for large sessile colorectal polyps (with video). Gastrointest Endosc 2012; 75(5):1086–91.
2. Committee AT, Hwang JH, Konda V, et al. Endoscopic mucosal resection. Gastrointest Endosc 2015;82(2):215–26.
3. Sethi A, Wong Kee Song LM. Adverse events related to colonic endoscopic mucosal resection and polypectomy. Gastrointest Endosc Clin N Am 2015; 25(1):55–69.
4. Luigiano C, Consolo P, Scaffidi MG, et al. Endoscopic mucosal resection for large and giant sessile and flat colorectal polyps: a single-center experience with long-term follow-up. Endoscopy 2009;41(10):829–35.
5. Burgess NG, Metz AJ, Williams SJ, et al. Risk factors for intraprocedural and clinically significant delayed bleeding after wide-field endoscopic mucosal resection of large colonic lesions. Clin Gastroenterol Hepatol 2014;12(4):651–61.e1-3.
6. Metz AJ, Bourke MJ, Moss A, et al. Factors that predict bleeding following endoscopic mucosal resection of large colonic lesions. Endoscopy 2011;43(6): 506–11.
7. Okano A, Hajiro K, Takakuwa H, et al. Predictors of bleeding after endoscopic mucosal resection of gastric tumors. Gastrointest Endosc 2003;57(6):687–90.
8. Fanning SB, Bourke MJ, Williams SJ, et al. Giant laterally spreading tumors of the duodenum: endoscopic resection outcomes, limitations, and caveats. Gastrointest Endosc 2012;75(4):805–12.
9. Park YM, Cho E, Kang HY, et al. The effectiveness and safety of endoscopic submucosal dissection compared with endoscopic mucosal resection for early gastric cancer: a systematic review and metaanalysis. Surg Endosc 2011; 25(8):2666–77.
10. Repici A, Hassan C, De Paula Pessoa D, et al. Efficacy and safety of endoscopic submucosal dissection for colorectal neoplasia: a systematic review. Endoscopy 2012;44(2):137–50.

11. Isomoto H, Yamaguchi N, Minami H, et al. Management of complications associated with endoscopic submucosal dissection/endoscopic mucosal resection for esophageal cancer. Dig Endosc 2013;25(Suppl 1):29–38.

12. Shin WG, Kim SJ, Choi MH, et al. Can rebamipide and proton pump inhibitor combination therapy promote the healing of endoscopic submucosal dissection-induced ulcers? A randomized, prospective, multicenter study. Gastrointest Endosc 2012;75(4):739–47.

13. Terasaki M, Tanaka S, Shigita K, et al. Risk factors for delayed bleeding after endoscopic submucosal dissection for colorectal neoplasms. Int J Colorectal Dis 2014;29(7):877–82.

14. Swan MP, Bourke MJ, Moss A, et al. The target sign: an endoscopic marker for the resection of the muscularis propria and potential perforation during colonic endoscopic mucosal resection. Gastrointest Endosc 2011;73(1):79–85.

15. Lian J, Chen S, Zhang Y, et al. A meta-analysis of endoscopic submucosal dissection and EMR for early gastric cancer. Gastrointest Endosc 2012;76(4):763–70.

16. Minami S, Gotoda T, Ono H, et al. Complete endoscopic closure of gastric perforation induced by endoscopic resection of early gastric cancer using endoclips can prevent surgery (with video). Gastrointest Endosc 2006;63(4):596–601.

17. Guo HM, Zhang XQ, Chen M, et al. Endoscopic submucosal dissection vs endoscopic mucosal resection for superficial esophageal cancer. World J Gastroenterol 2014;20(18):5540–7.

18. Zhang QS, Han B, Xu JH, et al. Clip closure of defect after endoscopic resection in patients with larger colorectal tumors decreased the adverse events. Gastrointest Endosc 2015;82(5):904–9.

19. Pohl H, Grimm IS, Moyer MT, et al. Clip closure prevents bleeding after endoscopic resection of large colon polyps in a randomized trial. Gastroenterology 2019. https://doi.org/10.1053/j.gastro.2019.03.019.

20. Matsuda T, Fujii T, Emura F, et al. Complete closure of a large defect after EMR of a lateral spreading colorectal tumor when using a two-channel colonoscope. Gastrointest Endosc 2004;60(5):836–8.

21. Wang J, Zhao L, Wang X, et al. A novel endoloop system for closure of colonic mucosal defects through a single-channel colonoscope. Endoscopy 2017;49(8):803–7.

22. Shi D, Li R, Chen W, et al. Application of novel endoloops to close the defects resulted from endoscopic full-thickness resection with single-channel gastroscope: a multicenter study. Surg Endosc 2017;31(2):837–42.

23. Abe S, Oda I, Mori G, et al. Complete endoscopic closure of a large gastric defect with endoloop and endoclips after complex endoscopic submucosal dissection. Endoscopy 2015;47(Suppl 1 UCTN):E374–5.

24. Akimoto T, Goto O, Nishizawa T, et al. Endoscopic closure after intraluminal surgery. Dig Endosc 2017;29(5):547–58.

25. Fujihara S, Mori H, Kobara H, et al. The efficacy and safety of prophylactic closure for a large mucosal defect after colorectal endoscopic submucosal dissection. Oncol Rep 2013;30(1):85–90.

26. Tashima T, Ohata K, Sakai E, et al. Efficacy of an over-the-scope clip for preventing adverse events after duodenal endoscopic submucosal dissection: a prospective interventional study. Endoscopy 2018;50(5):487–96.

27. Committee AT, Maple JT, Abu Dayyeh BK, et al. Endoscopic submucosal dissection. Gastrointest Endosc 2015;81(6):1311–25.

28. Draganov PV, Wang AY, Othman MO, et al. AGA institute clinical practice update: endoscopic submucosal dissection in the United States. Clin Gastroenterol Hepatol 2019;17(1):16–25.e1.
29. Kantsevoy SV, Bitner M, Mitrakov AA, et al. Endoscopic suturing closure of large mucosal defects after endoscopic submucosal dissection is technically feasible, fast, and eliminates the need for hospitalization (with videos). Gastrointest Endosc 2014;79(3):503–7.
30. Kantsevoy SV, Bitner M, Hajiyeva G, et al. Endoscopic management of colonic perforations: clips versus suturing closure (with videos). Gastrointest Endosc 2016;84(3):487–93.
31. Kantsevoy SV, Armengol-Miro JR. Endoscopic suturing, an essential enabling technology for new NOTES interventions. Gastrointest Endosc Clin N Am 2016; 26(2):375–84.
32. Han S, Wani S, Kaltenbach T, et al. Endoscopic suturing for closure of endoscopic submucosal dissection defects. VideoGIE 2019;4(7):310–3.

The Use of the Overstitch Beyond Bariatric Endoscopy
A Pictorial Description

Diego Juzgado, MD[a], Andres Sanchez-Yague, MD, PhD[b,c],*

KEYWORDS

- Endoscopic suture • Overstitch • Perforation • Fistula • Closure

KEY POINTS

- Endoscopic suturing may be used for defect closure, tissue compression, or as a traction or fixation method.
- Understanding suture patterns is important to unleash the full potential of the technique.
- Traction systems are not limited to the helicoidal device.

 Video content accompanies this article at http://www.giendo.theclinics.com.

The ability to suture through the endoscope has expanded the therapeutic capabilities of endoscopy. In this article, we present a comprehensive visual compendium to understand the concepts of endoscopic suturing in nonbariatric cases and to understand their potential applications. We focus our discussions on the currently widely available system, the Apollo Overstitch (Apollo Endosurgery, Austin, TX) (**Fig. 1**).

We describe the different types of suture patterns (**Figs. 2–12**). Then, we describe possible applications of the endoscopic suturing device, which include tissue compression without a defect, closure, traction, and fixation. Tissue compression without a defect refers mainly to bariatrics. The closure could be applied to perforations (**Figs. 13 and 14**), suture dehiscence (**Figs. 15 and 16**), fistulas (**Fig. 17**), and

Disclosure Statement: D. Juzgado: Consultant for Apollo Endosurgery. A. Sanchez-Yague: Nothing to disclose related to this article.
[a] Gastroenterology Department, Hospital Quironsalud Madrid, Madrid, Spain;
[b] Gastroenterology Department, Vithas Xanit International Hospital, Benalmadena, Spain;
[c] Interventinal Endoscopy, Gastroenterology Department, Hospital Costa del Sol, Autovia A-7, Km 187, Marbella 29603, Spain
* Corresponding author. Gastroenterology Department, Hospital Costa del Sol, Autovia A-7, Km 187, Marbella 29603, Spain.
E-mail address: asyague@gmail.com

giendo.theclinics.com

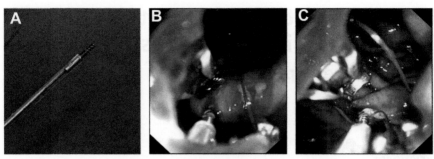

Fig. 1. The Apollo Overstitch system (Apollo Endosurgery, Austin, TX) uses a curved needle with a detachable tip at the end of a suture. The suture line is made of either absorbable and nonabsorbable material, although the nonabsorbable material is most commonly used. Once deployed, the detachable tip functions as a T-tag. To allow a deeper insertion of the needle, a traction method is used to pull the tissue toward the needle. The traction system is based mainly on the use of a corkscrew accessory (Tissue Helix, Apollo Endosurgery) (*A*). The corkscrew is pushed onto the mucosa and rotated for it to enters into the muscle layers. The corkscrew allows the wall to be pulled toward the needle with relative ease, although unscrewing the accessory can be challenging in some cases (*B*). Also, the line is prone to entanglement (*C*). Users are suggested to review and practice the use of the system in models. At the conclusions of stitching, the line is cinched detaching a fastener at the entry point where the first stitch entered the mucosa. (*Courtesy of* Apollo Endosurgery, Austin, TX.)

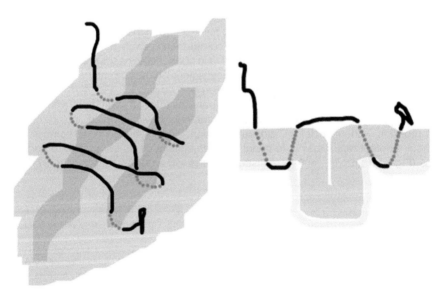

Fig. 2. Several suture patterns have been described, although not very well-studied.[1,2] (*Left*) In bariatric endoscopy, the most commonly used suture pattern is a variant of the inverted suture pattern, which is designed to compress the tissue together. (*Right*) Note that there is no wall defect to be approximated. The inverting suture pattern as applied using the endoscopic suturing system. This suture pattern is used in bariatric cases where there is no mucosal or wall defect. (*Courtesy of* Andres Sanchez-Yague, MD.)

Interrupted sutures

Direct   **Inverting**

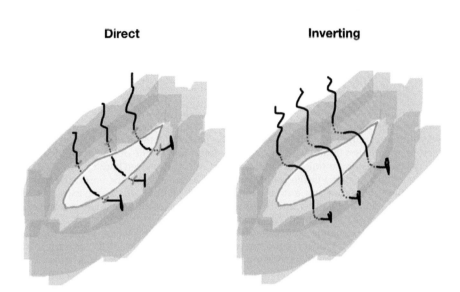

Fig. 3. Different suture patterns other than the variant of the inverted suture pattern are necessary to close a defect. We describe them according to the surgical descriptions. In surgery, the sutures could be interrupted or continuous (running) and they could be appositional, inverting or everting (**Fig. 4**). We describe the interrupted direct patterns using the endoscopic suturing system. (*Left*) In the direct interrupted suture, the line enters the mucosa exiting through the serosa, then passes underneath the mucosal defect and enters the serosa exiting through the mucosa. (*Right*) In the direct interrupted inverting suture, the line enters the mucosa passes through the serosa and exits the mucosa again, then passes over the mucosal defect finally enters the mucosa passes through the serosa and exits the mucosa again. (*Courtesy of* Andres Sanchez-Yague, MD.)

stoma reduction (**Fig. 18**). Traction could be applied either as a pulley method to improver resection (**Fig. 19**) or as an improved method to pull and, in turn, decrease a defect size and help pull it into an over the scope clips (**Fig. 20**). Fixation has been mainly used to secure endoluminal stents. Two stitching options are available: a direct suture that catches in the same stitch the wall and the stent and a hanging technique that stitches the wall, then the stent and finally the wall again (**Figs. 21–23**). The last technique allows a more comfortable removal because the line is better exposed, which in turn allows for easier access for cutting using the endoscopic scissors when the stent needs to be removed.

ACKNOWLEDGMENTS

The authors thank Dr Javier Valdes-Hernandez for his insights from a surgical point of view.

SUPPLEMENTARY DATA

Supplementary data related to this article can be found online at https://doi.org/10.1016/j.giec.2019.08.009.

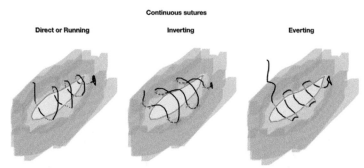

Fig. 4. The continuous suture patterns using the endoscopic suturing system. (*Left*) In the direct continuous suture (or running suture), the line enters the mucosa exiting through the serosa, then passes underneath the mucosal defect and on the other side of the defect enters the serosa exiting through the mucosa. The line is then moved back to the initial side for another stitch. (*Center*) In the continuous inverting suture, the line enters the mucosa passes through the serosa and exits the mucosa again on one side, then passes over the mucosal defect and on the other side enters the mucosa passes through the serosa and exits the mucosa again. The line is then moved back to the initial side for another stitch. (*Right*) The everting suture would be quite difficult to perform using the available endoscopic suturing system because it would require the whole system to be turned 180° on each stitch. Mainly, in this case, the line enters the mucosa on 1 side exiting through the serosa, then passes underneath the mucosal defect and on the other side of the defect enters the serosa exiting through the mucosa, then on the same side the line enters the mucosa exiting through the serosa, passes underneath the mucosal defect back to the initial side, where it enters the serosa exiting through the mucosa. (*Courtesy of* Andres Sanchez-Yague, MD.)

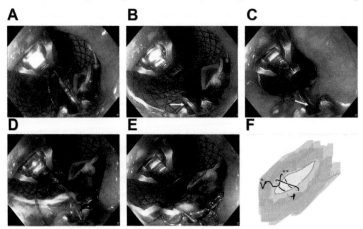

Fig. 5. Suture line trapped during stent fixation. It is essential to understand that the first stitch is the point where the line enters is the entry point where the fastener will need to be deployed to finish the suture. The line path leading to that entry point has to be clear meaning that we must avoid trapping it under the line on further stitches as otherwise the cinch may not be appropriately advanced toward the entry point creating loose sutures in some cases. The Suture line is trapped during stent fixation. Although it may look unusual, this disposition would allow for proper stitching as the trailing part of the line stays above the rest of the line (*A*). The line entry point can be seen through the stent (*white arrow*) (*B*). Moving the system toward the right side makes the subsequent stitch trap the trailing part of the line that leads to the entry point (*C*). The line traps the trailing part of the line. (*D, E*) This will hinder proper fastening of the suture because it will be difficult to approach the cinch to the entry point. In this schematic the trailing end (*asterisk*) that leads to the entry point (*double asterisks*) is trapped under the line after the second stitch (*F*). (*Courtesy of* [*A–E*] Apollo Endosurgery, Austin, TX; and [*F*] Andres Sanchez-Yague, MD.)

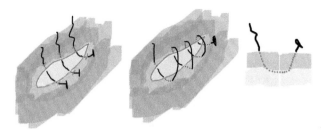

Direct sutures

Fig. 6. Direct sutures. Also referred to as apposing sutures achieve direct apposition of the tissues in the same plane. (*Courtesy of* Andres Sanchez-Yague, MD.)

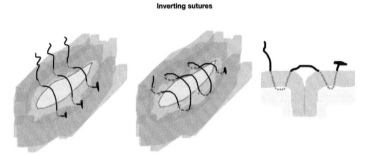

Inverting sutures

Fig. 7. Inverting sutures. Either interrupted or continuous turn incision edges inward confronting healthy mucosa. This suture pattern is not ideal for tissue healing. (*Courtesy of* Andres Sanchez-Yague, MD.)

Everting suture

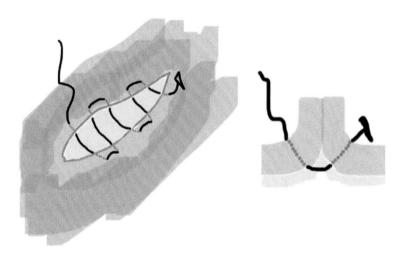

Fig. 8. Everting sutures turn the incision edges outwards. This suture pattern should improve tissue healing. However, although an everting suture creates even more apposition, it would require the endoscope to turn 180°, making it difficult to perform with the actual device. Future suturing device designs might make this suture pattern easier to perform. (*Courtesy of* Andres Sanchez-Yague, MD.)

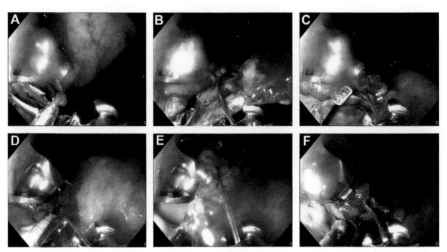

Fig. 9. A 2-step direct suture using a forceps. Direct sutures could be performed through a 2-step procedure or in a single step. A 2-step procedure would require grabbing 1 edge of the defect, stitch it from the mucosal to the serosal layer then grab the other edge and stitch it from the serosal to the mucosal layer. The forceps is opened to grab the edge of the defect (*A*). The stitch is seen crossing the mucosal side (*B*). The line emerges on the serosal side (*C*). The opposite edge is grabbed with the forceps (*D*). The opposite edge is moved toward the endoscope to allow stitching from the serosal to the mucosal side (*E*). In the end, the line enters the mucosal side on one edge exits it from the mucosal side on the other edge of the defect (*F*). (*Courtesy of* Apollo Endosurgery, Austin, TX.)

Incongruent apposition

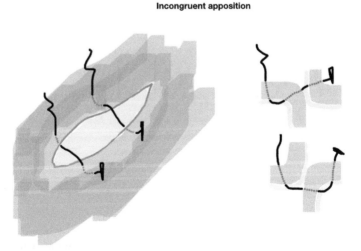

Fig. 10. Incongruent apposition. Creating the right suture pattern is important to achieve efficacious tissue apposition and prevent incongruent apposition. Abnormal apposition of mucosa toward serosa and vice versa can result from performing inconsistent stitching patterns in every edge of the incision. (*Courtesy of* Andres Sanchez-Yague, MD.)

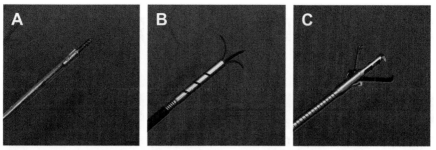

Fig. 11. Examples of currently available traction systems. Corkscrew traction system (Tissue Helix, Apollo Endosurgery, Austin, TX) (*A*). Triple-spiked retractable anchor system (Anchor, Ovesco Endoscopy AG, Tübingen, Germany) (*B*). Double opening grasping forceps (Twin Grasper, Ovesco Endoscopy AG) (*C*). The corkscrew traction system is most useful for creating the sleeves in bariatric endoscopy. However, when a defect is present, we have successfully used 2 additional traction methods: the Anchor, which allows more rooted, more stable, faster method to pull the wall (**Figs. 12** and **16**); or the standard single (**Fig. 9**) opening or the dual opening forceps (**Fig. 13**, Video 1). Alternatively, grabbing the corner of a perforation would also allow a single-step direct suture to be performed (**Fig. 15**). In other cases, when the edges are properly arranged suturing without a traction system may be possible (**Fig. 14**). (*Courtesy of* [*A*] Apollo Endosurgery, Austin, TX; and [*B*] Ovesco Endoscopy AG, Tübingen, Germany; and [*C*] Ovesco Endoscopy AG.)

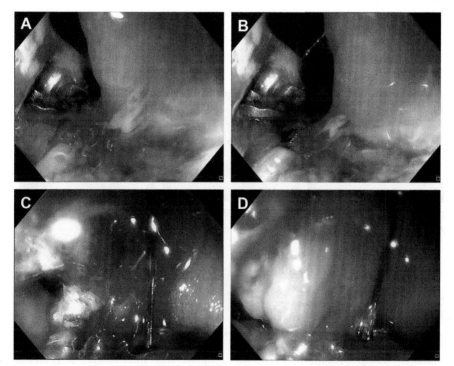

Fig. 12. Comparing the corkscrew traction system and the triple-spiked anchor. The corkscrew catheter faces the wall tangentially (*A*). After exiting the catheter, the corkscrew is rotated, but instead of digging into the mucosa, it slides over it (*B*). The triple-spiked device faces the mucosa in a similar position (*C*; Ovesco Endoscopy AG, Tübingen, Germany). Upon exiting the catheter, the spikes dig into the mucosa that is engaged and pulled toward the Overstitch (*D*). (*Courtesy of* Apollo Endosurgery, Austin, TX.)

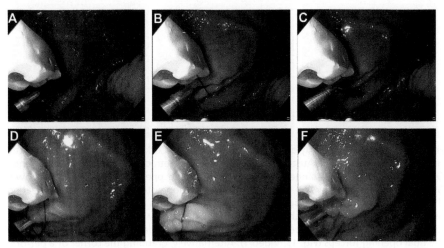

Fig. 13. Single-step running suture using a double opening forceps. One of the forceps arms is opened (*A*). The upper edge is grabbed (*B*). The other arm is opened to grab the lower edge (*C*). The tissue is pulled toward system (*D*). The tissue is stitched. (*E*). A single stitch passes both edges (*F*). This technique looks especially useful for defects with close edges owing to the difficulty to maneuver the double opening grasper after the first edge is grabbed. (*Courtesy of* Apollo Endosurgery, Austin, TX; and Ovesco Endoscopy AG, Tübingen, Germany.)

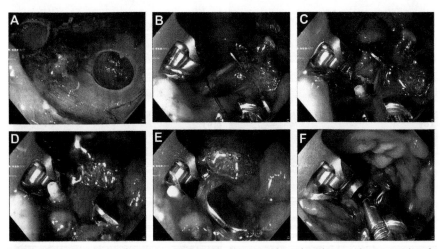

Fig. 14. Direct interrupted suturing without traction combined with over the scope clips for multiple perforations. In this case, 2 perforations were present after endoscopic mucosal resection of a large duodenal polyp (*A*). The first perforation was managed using an over the scope clips with including both perforations in the clip was not possible. Owing to the difficulty of positioning a second over the scope clips, suturing was attempted. Given the tangential approach, a direct interrupted suturing without a traction system was performed (*B*). The first stitch is fastened (*C*). To achieve deeper stitching, the system is pressed toward the defect (*D, E*). A second stitch is fastened (*F*), creating 2 interrupted direct sutures. ([*B–F*] *Courtesy of* Apollo Endosurgery, Austin, TX.)

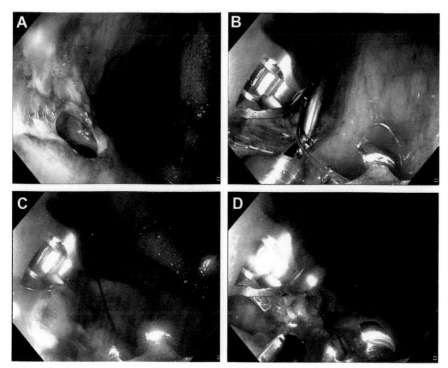

Fig. 15. Single-step running suture using a forceps. A suture dehiscence is visible (*A*). The defect corner is grabbed with the forceps (*B*) and pulled toward the Overstitch device (*C*). A single step direct suture is performed (*D*). ([*B–D*] *Courtesy of* Apollo Endosurgery, Austin, TX; and Ovesco Endoscopy AG, Tübingen, Germany.)

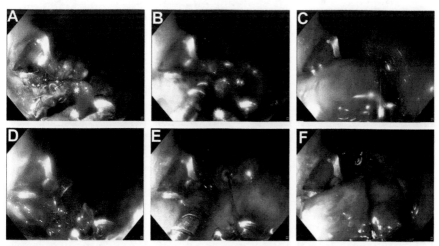

Fig. 16. Closing a dehiscence with the triple-spiked anchor creating a running 2-step suture. The staple line dehiscence can be seen (*A*). Securing the farther edge with the triple spiked anchor (*B*). Pulling the edge to stitch the tissue (*C*). The line enters the mucosal side and exits though the serosal side (*D*). The closest edge is grabbed with the anchor device (*E*). The tissue is stitched form the serosal side toward the mucosal side (*F*) creating a 2-step direct suture. (*Courtesy of* [*A, C, D, F*] Apollo Endosurgery, Austin, TX; and [*B, E*] Apollo Endosurgery, Austin, TX and Ovesco Endoscopy AG, Tübingen, Germany.)

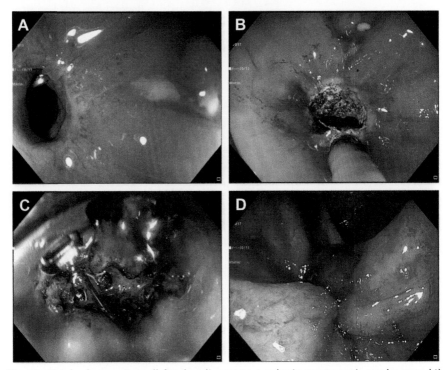

Fig. 17. Fistula closure. A small fistula adjacent to a colonic anastomosis can be seen (*A*). Ablation of the fistula edges with argon plasma is performed to facilitate closure during the healing process (*B*). Stitches are passed on both edges using a direct running suture (*C*) to close the defect (*D*). ([*C*] *Courtesy of* Apollo Endosurgery, Austin, TX.)

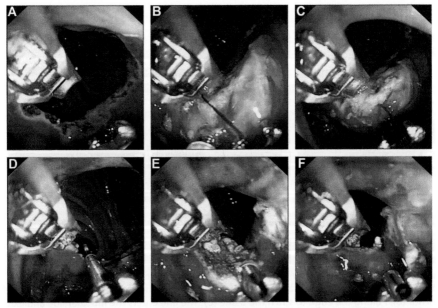

Fig. 18. Stoma closure. Enlargement of gastrojejunal anastomoses was found in this patient after surgery. Ablation of the stoma edges with argon plasma was performed to facilitate closure during the healing process (*A*). Stitches were placed in 2 different areas using a helicoidal traction system (*B, C*). Decrease of the stoma can be noted during the cinching process (*D, E*). The difference in stoma size is notable (*F*). (*Courtesy of* Apollo Endosurgery, Austin, TX.)

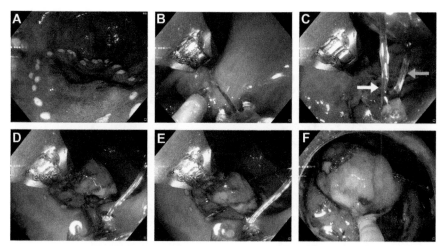

Fig. 19. Suture pulley method assisted endoscopic submucosal dissection. A gastric lesion was first marked before endoscopic submucosal dissection (*A*).[1] An area of the wall opposite to the lesion is selected to create the pulley. That area is moved toward the suturing system for the first stitch using the helicoidal device (*B*). It is important to note that the entry point (*white arrow*) should be proximal and the exiting point (green *arrow*) distal to allow for a proper run of the line during traction (*C*). The lesion is then stitched in the proximal margin to allow traction during endoscopic submucosal dissection (*D, E*). Pulling the line elevates the lesion and facilitates resection (*F*). ([*B–F*] *Courtesy of* Apollo Endosurgery, Austin, TX.)

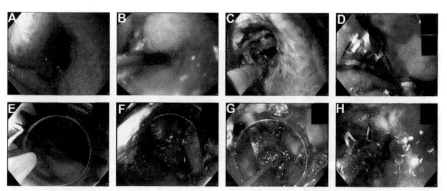

Fig. 20. Using a suture as a traction system to place an over the scope clips. A fistula with enlarged borders was found (*A*). The borders are too thick to be grabbed with a double opening forceps (*B*). Ablation of the fistula edges with argon plasma is performed to facilitate closure during the healing process (*C*). Several stitches are placed around the fistula edges (*D*). The double channel endoscope is removed, leaving the suture open. The suture is backloaded using a snare onto a regular endoscope with an over the scope clips fitted on the tip (*E*). The line is used to exert traction and pull the fistula into the over the scope clips cap (*F*). The line can be seen emerging from the middle of the over the scope clips after deployment (*G*). The suture is fastened (*H*) (Video 2). (*Courtesy of* [*B*] Ovesco Endoscopy AG, Tübingen, Germany; and [*D*] Apollo Endosurgery, Austin, TX; and [*E–H*] Apollo Endosurgery, Austin, TX and Ovesco Endoscopy AG, Tübingen, Germany.)

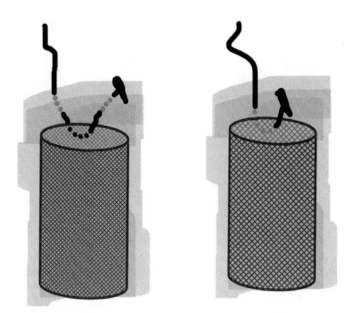

Fig. 21. Stent fixation options. In the "hanging" technique, first the wall is stitched, then the stent and finally the wall again (*left*). The direct suture that catches in the same stitch the wall and the stent (*right*). (*Courtesy of* Andres Sanchez-Yague, MD.)

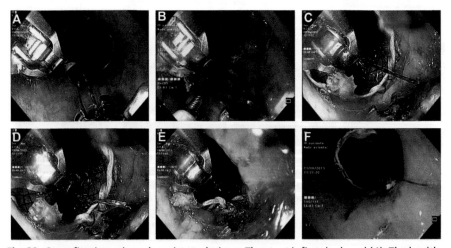

Fig. 22. Stent fixation using a hanging technique. The stent is first deployed (*A*). The healthy mucosa is stitched above the stent (*B*). The stent is stitched (*C*) but not the wall (*D*). The healthy mucosa is stitched above the stent (*E*). The stent is left hanging from the wall (*F*). (*Courtesy of* Apollo Endosurgery, Austin, TX.)

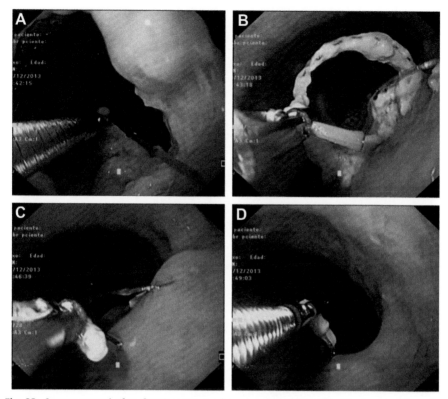

Fig. 23. Stent removal after fixation using a hanging technique. The line is cut with endoscopic scissors (*A*). The stent is pulled out using the removal line (*B*). The needle tip is removed with a forceps (*C*). The fastener is removed with a forceps (*D*).

REFERENCES

1. Stavropoulos SN, Modayil R, Friedel D. Current applications of endoscopic suturing. World J Gastrointest Endosc 2015;7(8):777–89.
2. Halvax P, Diana M, Nagao Y, et al. Experimental evaluation of the optimal suture pattern with a flexible endoscopic suturing system. Surg Innov 2017;24(3):201–4.

Complications of the Use of the OverStitch Endoscopic Suturing System

Jessica X. Yu, MD, MS*, Allison R. Schulman, MD, MPH

KEYWORDS

- Complications • Endoscopic suturing • OverStitch • Endoscopy

KEY POINTS

- OverStitch device can be safely used for a variety of indications.
- Providers should fully understand the OverStitch device as well as common trouble-shooting techniques to minimize the risk of complications.
- A clear understanding of the nuances of OverStitch use based on indication and tissue type is necessary.

INTRODUCTION

The OverStitch endoscopic suturing system (Apollo Endosurgery, Austin, TX) is a US Food and Drug Administration–cleared device for soft tissue approximation. It is a disposable, single-use, reloadable system that allows the placement of full-thickness sutures in a running or interrupted pattern without having to withdraw the endoscope. The original version of the device became available in 2008 but was simplified and re-released in 2011. Two iterations of this device are currently available. The OverStitch device requires a double-channel endoscope, and the newer OverStitch Sx is designed for compatibility with single-channel endoscopes.

Applications of endoscopic suturing are vast and include closure of partial-thickness or full-thickness defects, stent fixation, hemostasis and other management of ulcer disease, and bariatric procedures. The OverStitch system has been shown to be safe in experienced hands with minimal adverse events related to device use.[1] No specific immediate or delayed device-related complications have been reported in recent studies on the endoscopic closure of endoscopic submucosal dissection (ESD),[2] full-thickness defects,[3,4] stent fixation,[5] or for hemostasis.[6] Adverse outcomes are also infrequent after endoscopic sleeve gastroplasty, with recent studies reporting

Disclosure: None (J.X. Yu); Consultant for Boston Scientific, Microtech, Apollo Endosurgery (A. R. Schulman).
Division of Gastroenterology and Hepatology, University of Michigan, 1301 Catherine Street, Ann Arbor, MI 48109, USA
* Corresponding author. Division of Gastroenterology and Hepatology, Oregon Health and Sciences University, 3181 Southwest Sam Jackson Park Road, Mail Code: L461, Portland, OR 97239.
E-mail address: yujess@ohsu.edu

Gastrointest Endoscopy Clin N Am 30 (2020) 187–195
https://doi.org/10.1016/j.giec.2019.09.005
1052-5157/20/© 2019 Elsevier Inc. All rights reserved.

an overall adverse event rate of 2% to 5.2%.[7–12] These adverse events included perigastric fluid collections, leaks, intragastric and extragastric hemorrhage requiring blood transfusions, pneumoperitoneum, and pneumothorax.

The operation of the device can be cumbersome, and a thorough understanding of how to troubleshoot common device-related and procedure-related issues can help prevent complications and improve user efficiency. Although certain device-related complications are unique to the indication and planned procedure, this article focuses on common device-related complications and tips to prevent them.

DEVICE DESCRIPTION

The OverStitch device requires a double-channel endoscope (Olympus scopes GIF-2T160 or GIF-2T180; Olympus Corporation, Tokyo, Japan), with the distal attachment secured to the tip of the endoscope.[13] The recently released OverStitch Sx is designed for compatibility with single-channel endoscopes and is mounted using silicone straps distributed along the length of the catheter and end cap assembly.[14] The external catheter sheath has 2 working channels through which the OverStitch Sx accessories can be passed, independent of the endoscope channel. This article focuses primarily on the OverStitch device, because reported experience and existing data have evaluated this version.

The device consists of 3 components (**Fig. 1**)[13,15,16]:

- An end cap that houses a curved hollow needle body (see **Fig. 1**A)
- A needle driver handle that controls the opening and closing of the suture arm (see **Fig. 1**B)
- An anchor exchange (see **Fig. 1**C)

Additional accessories include the suture cassette, tissue helix, suture cinch, and overtube. The suture cassette contains the suture connected to a small tissue anchor, which also acts as both the tip of the suture needle and a T tag. Both absorbable (2-0, 3-0 polydioxanone) and non-absorbable sutures (2-0, 3-0 polypropylene) are available. The tissue helix can be used to acquire tissue by turning a rotating handle to advance a helical coil into the targeted area. The suture cinch is used to secure the suture in the final step of the procedure. By squeezing the handle, a polyetheretherketone (PEEK) cinch component is deployed onto the tail of the suture to secure it in place.

TECHNIQUE AND TROUBLESHOOTING
Preprocedure

Technique
The device is loaded by securing the end cap to the distal tip of the scope (see **Fig. 1**A). An anchor exchange, loaded with the suture, is then advanced into one of the working channels to the needle (see **Fig. 1**C). Stitches are made by passing the suture between the anchor exchange and the needle body.

Pitfalls and potential complications
Improper loading of the device before insertion can cause problems with device usage and result in the device breaking or not functioning during the procedure, necessitating withdrawing the scope or replacing the device.

Tips and troubleshooting

- Care should be taken to ensure the actuator cable travels straight along the scope shaft to ensure the hand controls operate the needle correctly.

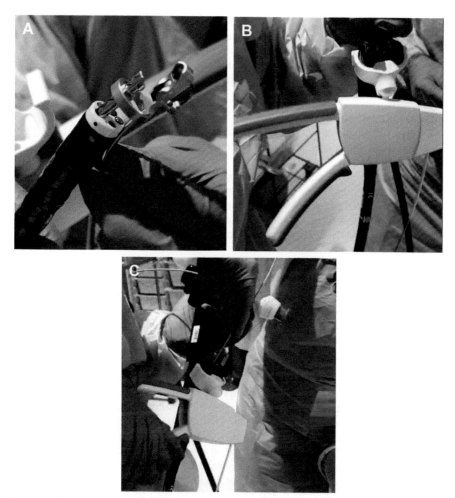

Fig. 1. Device components with end cap (*A*), needle driver handle (*B*), and anchor exchange (*C*).

- When loading the suture, the tip of the anchor exchange should be within the alignment tube to prevent needle bending with the closure of the needle driver handle.
- The anchor exchange loaded with the suture should be passed beyond the alignment tube several times to create slack and minimize tension on the suture.
- A full cycle of loading and unloading the suture should be performed before insertion of the loaded device to minimize troubleshooting during the procedure.

Intraprocedure

Scope passage and device maneuvering
Technique The scope loaded with the OverStitch device should be carefully advanced with the needle in the closed position.

Pitfalls and potential complications The end cap assembly, especially with the needle open, increases both the length and width of the distal end of the scope. Safe passage of the OverStitch device is critical to avoid trauma and injury to the posterior oropharynx,[17] esophagus, and through areas of stenosis. An overtube is often used to facilitate passage of the device; however, mucosal trauma, lacerations, and even perforation have been reported with overtube placement.[18–20] In addition, the device can cause mucosal and luminal injury unless carefully maneuvered, especially in areas of thin or ulcerated tissue.

Tips and troubleshooting
- Never push against significant resistance.
- The needle driver should always be in the closed position before advancing the endoscope.
- Additional lubrication, scope torqueing, or repositioning of the patient's head or neck may be necessary for safe advancement.
- Use of an overtube should be considered to facilitate device passage.[18] Placement of the patient in a sword-swallower position with a jaw thrust during passage of the overtube may facilitate nontraumatic advancement.[18]

Suturing
Technique The target tissue is grasped with the tissue helix and pulled toward the scope. A full-thickness bite is made by passing the loaded needle through the target tissue by closing the needle driver handle. The needle is then passed onto the anchor exchange. Additional stitches can be made by reloading the needle and passing the suture between the needle body and anchor exchange. Single or multiple bites can be taken in various patterns without having to withdraw the scope.

Pitfalls and potential complications The success of the OverStitch device is largely caused by its ability to facilitate full-thickness sutures; partial-thickness bites decrease the durability of the sutures. Placement of sutures and patterns should be carefully selected based on the indication, because this may affect the durability of the sutures.[21] With more complex patterns, such as purse-string and running sutures, there is the potential for crossing and creating knots, which decrease the strength of the suture and hinder completion of the desired pattern. Prematurely dropping or breaking the suture could mean the loss of the entire suture.

The tissue helix is used to grasp tissue but can lead to bleeding and mucosal trauma. Perforation directly attributed to the use of the tissue helix during endoscopic sleeve gastroplasty has also been described.[22] The tissue helix could also potentially injure adjacent organs. Bleeding has also been reported with full-thickness suturing.[23]

Tips and troubleshooting
- To ensure full-thickness bites, the scope should be maneuvered toward the left as the tissue helix is being pulled toward the scope tip (**Fig. 2**).
- With more complex patterns, be aware of the location of the suture to prevent crossing sutures and knots.
- If the suture is prematurely dropped, the suture should be cinched immediately.
- Do not pull the suture into the scope during the cinching process until the suture has been cinched, because the attached T tag can lead to scope damage and inadequate suture tension.
- It is important to ensure that the tissue helix is carefully deployed and retracted to avoid trapping tissue and causing trauma. This maneuver can be accomplished by having the assistant count and keep track of each turn of the helix during deployment and retract with the same number of turns.

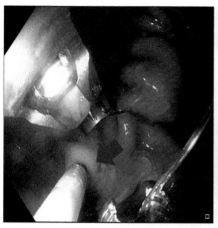 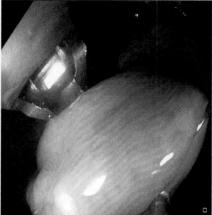

Fig. 2. Rolling the scope to the left as illustrated by the arrow in the left panel while the tissue helix is used to pull the target tissue toward the suturing device helps to ensure full-thickness bites as demonstrated in the right panel.

- To avoid deeper tissue injury, perforation, and injury to adjacent organs, it is important to avoid using excessive pressure or an excessive number of turns when deploying the helix.
- If significant bleeding is encountered during a full-thickness bite, the suture should be cinched immediately (**Fig. 3**).

Cinching
Technique Once the suture is completed, the needle is dropped away from the distal tip of the scope. A cinch is loaded onto the end of the suture and advanced to the tissue. The suture is slowly tightened and the cinch is deployed.

Pitfalls and potential complications The suture should be dropped away from the tip of the scope because the T tag can damage the scope channel. The suture should be carefully tightened against the cinch; tightening the suture excessively may cause suture breakage and loss of the suture.

Tips and troubleshooting
- After the suture pattern is completed, the needle should be dropped 3 cm from the tip of the scope to avoid damaging the scope (**Fig. 4**A, B).
- Long, slow pulls of the suture before deploying the cinch can help tighten the suture.
- The cinch should be held straight near the first stitch that was placed to avoid breaking the cinch (**Fig. 4**C–E).
- The cinch should be deployed by closing the handle with both hands until a click is noted. Further closing the handle at this point can break the cinch.

Postprocedure

Scope withdrawal
Technique Once the suture is cinched and the procedure completed, the device handle should be closed and carefully withdrawn. The overtube, if used, should be carefully removed. The mucosa should be inspected for any trauma.

Pitfalls and potential complications Similar to insertion, withdrawing the device with the needle in the open position may cause luminal injury.

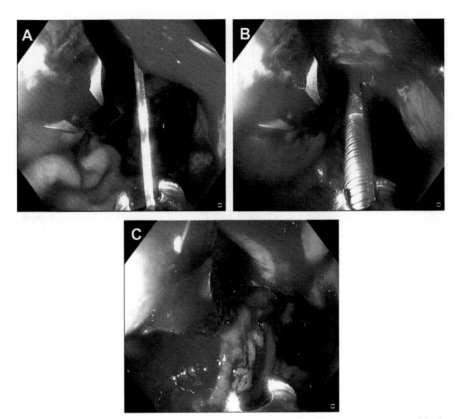

Fig. 3. Bleeding is encountered after taking a full-thickness bite (*A*). A cinch was quickly deployed (*B*), after which the bleeding resolved (*C*).

Tips and troubleshooting
- Ensure the needle is closed before withdrawing the scope.
- Carefully inspect the mucosa on withdrawal and after removal of the overtube for any trauma that may require treatment.

Delayed complications
Techniques The patient should be carefully monitored after the procedure for any signs of delayed postprocedure complications.

Pitfalls and potential complications Recent studies have reported no significant delayed device-related complications with the use of the OverStitch for stent fixation, closure of defects, stomal revision, or hemostasis.[1–6] Delayed complications after endoscopic sleeve gastroplasty are also rare, with rates of perigastric fluid collections ranging from 0.4% to 2.3%.[7–9,11,12] Treatment may require drainage and antibiotics. Other complications, such as delayed bleeding, pneumoperitoneum, pneumothorax, and perforation,[24] have also been reported but, again, are rare. Complications such as perigastric fluid collections and bleeding have been attributed to suturing of the gastric fundus, which has a thin wall and is adjacent to the spleen.[25,26] The risk of complications can similarly be extrapolated to other areas of thin-walled tissue.

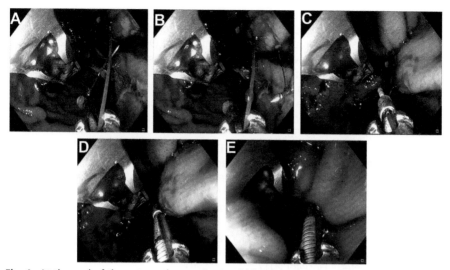

Fig. 4. At the end of the suture, the needle should be dropped away from the scope tip (*A,* *B*). The cinch is advanced over the suture and should be kept in a straight position while the suture is tightened (*C–E*).

Tips and techniques
- Care should be applied when suturing in areas of thin-walled tissue.
- Patients should receive clear and detailed postprocedural instructions. Medication modifications, such as starting proton pump inhibitors or holding anticoagulation, should be discussed, and follow-up plans should be arranged.

SUMMARY

Endoscopic suturing with the OverStitch system is a safe technique with many applications. Device-related complications are rare. Successful use of the OverStitch system requires not only an understanding of the device but also awareness of potential pitfalls and complications that may be unique to the intended procedure. Increased cognizance of tips and troubleshooting techniques helps minimize potential adverse events.

REFERENCES

1. Yang J, Lee D, Siddiqui A. Current developments in endoscopic suturing. Pract Gastroenterol 2015;39(10):9.
2. Kantsevoy SV, Bitner M, Mitrakov AA, et al. Endoscopic suturing closure of large mucosal defects after endoscopic submucosal dissection is technically feasible, fast, and eliminates the need for hospitalization (with videos). Gastrointest Endosc 2014;79(3):503–7.
3. Kantsevoy SV, Bitner M, Hajiyeva G, et al. Endoscopic management of colonic perforations: clips versus suturing closure (with videos). Gastrointest Endosc 2016;84(3):487–93.
4. Kukreja K, Chennubhotla S, Bhandari B, et al. Closing the gaps: endoscopic suturing for large submucosal and full-thickness defects. Clin Endosc 2018;51(4): 352–6.

5. Ngamruengphong S, Sharaiha R, Sethi A, et al. Fully-covered metal stents with endoscopic suturing vs. partially-covered metal stents for benign upper gastrointestinal diseases: a comparative study. Endosc Int Open 2018;6(2):E217–23.

6. Agarwal A, Benias P, Brewer Gutierrez OI, et al. Endoscopic suturing for management of peptic ulcer-related upper gastrointestinal bleeding: a preliminary experience. Endosc Int Open 2018;6(12):E1439–44.

7. Lopez-Nava G, Sharaiha RZ, Vargas EJ, et al. Endoscopic Sleeve gastroplasty for obesity: a multicenter study of 248 patients with 24 months follow-up. Obes Surg 2017;27(10):2649–55.

8. Barrichello S, Hourneaux de Moura DT, Hourneaux de Moura EG, et al. Endoscopic sleeve gastroplasty in the management of overweight and obesity: an international multicenter study. Gastrointest Endosc 2019. [Epub ahead of print].

9. Alqahtani A, Al-Darwish A, Mahmoud AE, et al. Short-term outcomes of endoscopic sleeve gastroplasty in 1000 consecutive patients. Gastrointest Endosc 2019;89(6):1132–8.

10. Sharaiha RZ, Kumta NA, Saumoy M, et al. Endoscopic sleeve gastroplasty significantly reduces body mass index and metabolic complications in obese patients. Clin Gastroenterol Hepatol 2017;15(4):504–10.

11. Fayad L, Cheskin LJ, Adam A, et al. Endoscopic sleeve gastroplasty versus intragastric balloon insertion: efficacy, durability, and safety. Endoscopy 2019;51(6):532–9.

12. Fayad L, Adam A, Schweitzer M, et al. Endoscopic sleeve gastroplasty versus laparoscopic sleeve gastrectomy: a case-matched study. Gastrointest Endosc 2019;89(4):782–8.

13. Parsi MA, Schulman AR, Aslanian HR, et al. Devices for endoscopic hemostasis of nonvariceal GI bleeding (with videos). VideoGIE 2019;4(7):285–99.

14. OverStitch SX™ Endoscopic Suturing System. 2019. Available at: https://www.overstitch.com/overstitch-sx. Accessed August 1, 2019.

15. Banerjee S, Barth BA, Bhat YM, et al. Endoscopic closure devices. Gastrointest Endosc 2012;76(2):244–51.

16. Weilert F, Binmoeller KF. New endoscopic technologies and procedural advances for endoscopic hemostasis. Clin Gastroenterol Hepatol 2016;14(9):1234–44.

17. Stavropoulos SN, Modayil R, Friedel D. Current applications of endoscopic suturing. World J Gastrointest Endosc 2015;7(8):777–89.

18. Storm AC, Vargas EJ, Matar R, et al. Esophageal overtubes provide no benefit to safety or technical success in upper gastrointestinal tract endoscopic suturing. Endosc Int Open 2019;7(7):E919–21.

19. Tierney WM, Adler DG, Conway JD, et al. Overtube use in gastrointestinal endoscopy. Gastrointest Endosc 2009;70(5):828–34.

20. Vargas EJ, Bazerbachi F, Rizk M, et al. Transoral outlet reduction with full thickness endoscopic suturing for weight regain after gastric bypass: a large multicenter international experience and meta-analysis. Surg Endosc 2018;32(1):252–9.

21. Schulman AR, Huseini M, Thompson CC. Endoscopic sleeve gastroplasty of the remnant stomach in Roux-en-Y gastric bypass: a novel approach to a gastrogastric fistula with weight regain. Endoscopy 2018;50(6):E132–3.

22. Saumoy M, Schneider Y, Zhou XK, et al. A single-operator learning curve analysis for the endoscopic sleeve gastroplasty. Gastrointest Endosc 2018;87(2):442–7.

23. Hill C, El Zein M, Agnihotri A, et al. Endoscopic sleeve gastroplasty: the learning curve. Endosc Int Open 2017;5(9):E900–4.

24. Surve A, Cottam D, Medlin W, et al. A video case report of gastric perforation following endoscopic sleeve gastroplasty and its surgical treatment. Obes Surg 2019. [Epub ahead of print].
25. de Moura DTH, de Moura EGH, Thompson CC. Endoscopic sleeve gastroplasty: from whence we came and where we are going. World J Gastrointest Endosc 2019;11(5):322–8.
26. James TW, McGowan CE. The descending gastric fundus in endoscopic sleeve gastroplasty: implications for procedural technique and adverse events. Video-GIE 2019;4(6):254–5.

Optimized Training in the Use of Endoscopic Closure Devices

Majidah Abdulfattah Bukhari, MD, FASGE, FRCPC, ABIM, MRCP (GI)[a,b],
Mouen A. Khashab, MD[a,c],*

KEYWORDS

- Endoscopic closure • Gastrointestinal perforation • Gastrointestinal Leak
- Gastrointestinal fistula • Devices • Techniques • Endoscopic management
- Advantages • Limitations

KEY POINTS

- There is no best technique that can be applied to close all gastrointestinal defects. The endoscopist must be familiar with different devices and techniques.
- Endoscopic closure is a minimally invasive therapy that is used as an alternative to surgical repair and can be achieved using a variety of devices.
- Proper training in endoscopic closure is mandatory to achieve successful results.
- Close collaboration with surgeons is important in the management of patients with gastrointestinal defects after endoscopic closure.
- Endoscopic clipping and suturing techniques are commonly used to close perforations.

INTRODUCTION

Gastrointestinal (GI) defects occur when there is disruption of the GI wall owing to various pathologies. GI defects are classified into 3 main entities: leaks, fistulae, and perforations. A leak is defined as an abnormal communication between the intraluminal and the extraluminal compartments. Leaks usually occur at sites of surgical anastomosis. A fistula is defined as an abnormal communication between 2 epithelized surfaces. A perforation is an acute, full-thickness defect of the GI wall.[1] The clinical presentation of each entity depends on the location of the defect, the nature of the

Financial Disclosures and Conflicts of Interest: M. A. Khashab is a consultant and on medical advisory board for Boston Scientific and Olympus and a consultant for Medtronic.
a Division of Gastroenterology and Hepatology, Johns Hopkins Medical Institutions, Baltimore, MD, USA; b Division of Medicine and Gastroenterology and Hepatology, International Medical Center, Jeddah 23214, Saudi Arabia; c Division of Gastroenterology and Hepatology, Johns Hopkins Hospital, 1800 Orleans Street, Zayed Building, Suite 7125B, Baltimore, MD 21287, USA
* Corresponding author. Division of Gastroenterology and Hepatology, Johns Hopkins Hospital, 1800 Orleans Street, Zayed Bldg, Suite 7125B, Baltimore, MD 21287.
E-mail address: mkhasha1@jhmi.edu

Gastrointest Endoscopy Clin N Am 30 (2020) 197–208
https://doi.org/10.1016/j.giec.2019.08.008
1052-5157/20/© 2019 Elsevier Inc. All rights reserved.

contents of the intraluminal compartment, and the anatomic relationship with adjacent organs. The greatest cause for concern is the spilling of GI contents and bacteria into the sterile intra-abdominal or intrathoracic cavities, which may lead to serious systemic inflammation and infection. Thus, early detection and prompt therapy are crucial for a favorable outcome.

In recent years, there has been a paradigm shift in the management of GI defects, especially with the development of various endoscopic closure devices. The principle of management of GI defects is the prevention of luminal leakage by endoscopic closure with either endoscopic clips, sutures, or by diversion of the contents using endoscopic stenting. Learning how to close a GI lesion will aid endoscopists in avoiding the need for surgical repair. The ideal closure device should be effective, safe, inexpensive, and easy to use. It should also be robust and durable.

In this article, we highlight available endoscopic devices (mainly endoscopic clipping and suturing) and the techniques used to close GI defects.

THE REQUIRED SKILL SET

The trainee should be familiar with the use and operation of different closure devices and know how and when to use each device based on the various clinical scenarios. The trainee should learn the necessary skills by performing clinical cases under direct supervision of an expert endoscopist, which allows for real-time personal feedback. Maintaining and honing these skills by the regular use of closure devices is essential. Encouraging the trainee to read, attend live endoscopy courses, workshops, videos and interactive teaching programs, and practicing on live animal models will help the trainee to recognize and understand the different devices available and expand their knowledge.

Required Knowledge and Technical Skills to Be Mastered by the Trainee Before Learning Endoscopic Closure

1. Sound knowledge of basic endoscopic skills.
2. Knowledge of all endoscopic devices, their application, and limitations during endoscopic closure.
3. Be cautious and gentle with the use of the endoscope and any endoscopic instruments.
4. Be calm and comfortable working in a controlled environment.
5. A good working relationship with an experienced endoscopic assistant is crucial.
6. Good communication skills are mandatory for proper and coordinated use of the devices.
7. Identification and proper assessment of the GI defects.
8. Awareness of endoscopic and nonendoscopic management for GI defects.
9. Learn how to carry out urgent decompression in case of complications such as pneumothorax or pneumoperitoneum.
10. Learn how to deliver the device around the defect in a controlled manner.
11. Carbon dioxide (CO_2) should always be used during prolonged procedures because it is absorbed much faster than air.
12. Avoid aggressive air insufflation because this maneuver will stretch the wall of the gut and increase the size of the defect. It also increases the risk of pneumoperitoneum or pneumothorax and may worsen the patient's cardiopulmonary status.
13. Avoid overinflation and decompress the lumen before withdrawing the endoscope.
14. Postoperative care is a part of successful outcomes.

MANAGEMENT OF GASTROINTESTINAL DEFECTS

Endoscopic closure of GI defects can be achieved using a variety of endoscopic tools. In some cases, concomitant use of more than one device is necessary to achieve a desired clinical response. Each device has a different technique and closure mechanism, with its own advantages and disadvantages. Currently, no data can definitely recommend one technique over another; the endoscopist should be aware of local expertise and availability of endoscopic tools, and on-site surgical backup before attempting any challenging cases.

ENDOSCOPIC CLOSURE DEVICES
Through the Scope Clips

Through the scope clips (TTSCs; also known as endoclips) were first introduced to achieve endoscopic hemostasis. Nowadays, they are also being used to close GI defects less than 2 cm in size, with a success rate ranging from 59% to 83%.[2–5] TTSCs are widely available, easy to use, and can rotate and reopen if required.

Characteristics of through the scope clips

TTSC devices are made of 2 components: metallic pronged clips and a delivery catheter handle that are introduced through the working channel of the endoscope. The clips come in multiple sizes, different lengths and width spans, rotation capacities, and deployments after multiple openings. The rotating mechanism is important for precise deployment in a correct direction. All TTSCs fit through the standard working channel (2.8 mm) of a gastroscope, and are available for all types of endoscopes.

Commercially available through the scope clips

TTSCs are relatively similar, and the use of one clip over the other depends on availability and personal preference:

1. The QuickClip2 and QuickClip2 long (Olympus America Inc, Center Valley, PA) can open, close, and reopen with 360° rotation (1:1). The QuickClip2 long is longer than QuickClip2 to allow grasping of more tissue. The width of the open jaw of the clip is either 9 or 11 mm (**Fig. 1**A, B).
2. The Resolution Clip and Resolution 360 Clip (Boston Scientific Inc, Natick, MA). The Resolution 360 Clip has 1:1 rotation and can reopen after closure for reposition, if required. It has an open width of 11 mm (**Fig. 1**C, D).
3. The Instinct Endoscopic Hemoclip (Cook Medical, Bloomington, IN). The clip is rotatable through 360°, and can reopen for reposition. It has an open width of 16 mm (**Fig. 1**E).
4. The DuraClip Repositional Clip (ConMed Corporation, Utica, NY), comes in a width of either 11 or 16 mm, with 1:1 rotation and can open and close for an unlimited number of times before deployment (**Fig. 1**F).
5. The SureClip (Micro-Tech, Nanjing, China), which is a rotatable clip, comes in 3 widths: 8, 11, and 16 mm (**Fig. 1**G).

Through the scope clip application technique

Advance the closed clip through the working channel to the site of interest, and ask your assistant to open the device jaws. Keep the open clip close to the end of the endoscope to be able to manipulate the clip-endoscope as one unit. The open clip is oriented (either through manipulation of the endoscope shaft or by rotating the clip apparatus) perpendicular to the axis of the lesion. Engage the lower jaw to the lower edge of the defect, and gently push the scope-clip unit. At the same time, gently apply suction to collapse the lumen and allow the opposite edge of

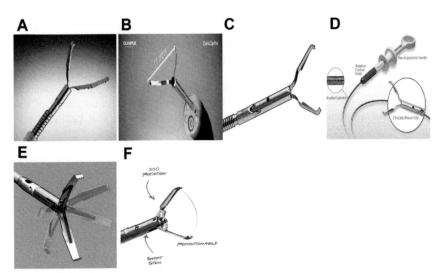

Fig. 1. (*A*) QuickClip2. (*B*) QuickClip2 long. (*C*) Resolution clip. (*D*) Resolution 360 Clip. (*E*) Instinct Endoscopic Hemoclip. (*F*) DuraClip Repositional Clip. (*G*) SureClip. ([*A, B*] *Courtesy of* Olympus America Inc, Center Valley, PA; [*C, D*] *Courtesy of* Boston Scientific Inc., Natick, MA; [*E*] *Courtesy of* Cook Medical, Bloomington, IN; [*F*] *Courtesy of* Micro-Tech, Nanjing, China; with permission.)

the defect to be grasped as deeply as possible while slowly closing the clip. Ensure satisfactory clip closure before deployment of the clip. The first clip is always the most critical one when it comes to closure of a defect, because it will tent the mucosal defect and make subsequent application of clips more effective and easier. Place any additional clips from top to bottom in linear defects, or left to right in circular defects. The number of the clips to be used to close a defect depends on the size of the lesion; for instance, a small defect that is, less than 5 mm, may need 3 clips, whereas a 10-mm defect may need 5 or more clips to achieve satisfactory closure.

Limitations of through the scope clips
TTSCs are effective in closing small lesions up to 2 cm in size; however, closure of a larger defect (>3 cm) using TTSCs might be unreliable. This is due to the restricted opening distance between the 2 jaws and the superficial closing force, which are insufficient to close beyond the superficial submucosa. Early detachment can occur because of the increased extension force.[6] In addition, closing a defect surrounded by inflamed or ulcerated mucosa may be more challenging with a TTSC.

Key points for successful endoscopic closure with through the scope clips
1. Be patient and careful when deploying the first clip. The first clip is the most critical aspect of a successful clip closure. Remember that a misplaced first clip might make the placement of additional clips technically difficult.
2. Avoid excessive movement while the clip is open because this may stretch the tissue and interfere with tissue approximation.
3. Keep the clip close to the end of the endoscope so that you will be able to manipulate both as a one unit.
4. Align the opened clip in the intended position perpendicular to the defect.

5. Approach a linear defect from above and deploy the first clip just above the upper end of the linear defect. This maneuver will tent the tissue up for easier application of subsequent clips from the top down.
6. Approach a circular defect from below or from left to right with intended transverse closure.
7. Gently push the unit while applying suction before closing the clip to approximate both edges of the lesion.
8. Confirm satisfactory clip closure with edge-to-edge approximation before deploying the clip; failure to do so will interfere with complete tissue approximation.
9. Steadily release the clip after deployment and detach it from the clip deployment catheter to avoid it acting as a biopsy forceps when being withdrawn from the endoscope channel.
10. The delivery system should be introduced carefully without dislodging any clips.
11. Tension pneumoperitoneum requires prompt decompression using a large-bore needle puncture of the peritoneal cavity. In case of acute perforation, the procedure can be carried out without removing the endoscope. Once tension pneumoperitoneum is relieved, the defect can then be closed endoscopically.

Over the scope Clips

Over the scope clips are able to close large defects up to 3 cm in size (US Food and Drug Administration clearance has been obtained for luminal perforation closure of <2 cm in size).[7] Over the scope clips are more durable and can reliably close full-thickness defects.[8,9] In defects larger than 2 cm, the deployment of 2 adjacent clips has been reported.[10] The over the scope clips devices have wider clip arms, which enable them to grasp more tissue within the cap and with greater force.[8]

Types of the over the scope clips

1. Ovesco Endoscopy AG (Tübingen, Germany) (**Fig. 2**)
2. Padlock-G clip (US Endoscopy, Mentor, OH) (**Fig. 3**)

The Padlock-G clip has a similar principle to the Ovesco. The Padlock clip has a catheter that runs parallel to the insertion tube of the endoscope and is attached to a syringe-like trigger, which deployed the clips.

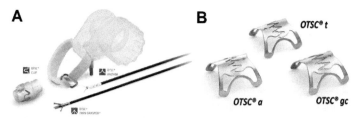

Fig. 2. (*A*) The over the scope clips System. (*B*) Type of over the scope clips (Ovesco): (*a-type*) A-clip with blunt teeth (*round*) that is primarily used for hemostasis. (*t-type*) T-clip with short sharp teeth (*pointed*) that is used for defect closure in indurated or fibrotic area to decrease the risk of clip detachment. (*gc type*) Gastric clip with long sharper teeth (long pointer) that is used for full-thickness gastric defects. (*Courtesy of* Ovesco Endoscopy AG, Tubingen, Germany; with permission.)

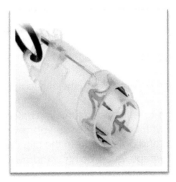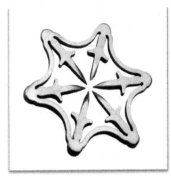

Fig. 3. Padlock clip defect closure system. (*Courtesy of* US Endoscopy, Mentor, OH; with permission.)

Characteristics of the over the scope clips The over the scope clips system includes an applicator cap, a clip, and a handle (wheel) (see **Fig. 2**A). The over the scope clips is super-elastic nitinol with teeth arranged like a bear trap (in the open position), that fits over a distal clear cap at the end of the endoscope and is connected to a wheel by a string for releasing the clip. The mechanism for deployment is similar to that used for band ligation. The wheel is attached to the working channel of the endoscope. The clip is released to the target site by turning the wheel clockwise until a click is felt. There are 3 types of over the scope clips devices (see **Fig. 2**B).

The caps are available in 3 sizes to accommodate a variety of endoscope diameters:

1. The 11-mm device is designed for endoscope diameters ranging from 9.5 to 11.0 mm.
2. The 12-mm device is for endoscope diameters ranging from 10.5 to 12.0 mm.
3. The 14-mm device is for endoscope diameters ranging from 11.5 to 14.0 mm.

The corresponding outer diameters of the caps attached to the endoscope are 16.5 mm, 17.5 mm, and 21.0 mm, respectively. There are 2 depth of caps (3 and 6 mm) to allow tissue grasping during approximation.

- *Aid instruments*: Three aid instruments are available to facilitate the use with the over the scope clips whenever needed:
  - *Twin grasper:* This allows the endoscopist to sequentially grasp the opposite edges of the defect and separately and pull them to approximate the tissue before deployment of the clip. This device is used when the defect is large and the suction method is insufficient to grasp tissue. The instrument has 2 independent jaws that can be opened to grasp the tissue into the cap.
  - *Anchor:* The anchor device has 3 retractable needle pins to anchor and pull the fibrotic tissue and ulcer into the cap when the suction method and twin grasper are unable to grasp the tissue. After deploying the clip, the anchor is then retracted and removed.
  - *Reloader:* This is a device that assists in mounting additional clips onto the applicator cap after placement of the first over the scope clips, in case more than 1 clip is needed to close the defect.

Over the Scope Clips closure technique

Deployment of an over the scope clips is simple and straightforward; yet, it is important to follow the steps carefully for a successful outcome. After assessment of the defect, the endoscope is withdrawn from the patient. The hand wheel (yellow) is attached to the working channel. The applicator cap with a preloaded clip is then attached to the tip of the endoscope similarly to a band ligator using a thread retriever. The clip release thread is pulled retrogradely through the working channel of the scope and fixed onto a hand wheel. The endoscope preloaded with the over the scope clips is then advanced to the site of interest. The over the scope clips is positioned at the target site (align the lesion in a 6–12 o'clock position). Using a simple suction method, the twin grasper, or the tissue anchor methods, is used to grasp both edges of the defect and pull them into the distal cap before placing the clip. The handle should be quickly turned in a clockwise direction to deploy the clip onto the target. One should avoid capturing the twin grasper by the clip.

Limitations of the Over the Scope Clips
The over the scope clips allows closure of larger lesions with greater closure force; however, in case of larger perforations requiring more than 1 clip, it is mandatory to withdraw the endoscope from the patient to assemble the clip. The other limitation is the size of the clip that may be difficult to advance into the oropharynx, upper esophageal sphincter, or through a narrowed or tortuous lumen. Deployment of an over the scope-clips is difficult in retroflex view or when the lesion is surrounded with inflamed or ulcerated mucosa.

Key points for successful endoscopic closure with an over the scope clips

1. Align the lesion in a 6 to 12 o'clock position as much as possible.
2. For small defects, the suction method may be enough to grasp the defect and the surrounding tissue into the distal cap before deployment of the over the scope clips.
3. Use a twin grasper or the anchor device to facilitate the use of the over the scope clips to close a large defect.
4. Pull the grasper with the tissue into the center of the distal cap to ensure that the entire lesion is within the cap.
5. The key element to successful closure is the position of the lesion within the over the scope-clips cap, as misplacement to one side of the defect can affect successful placement of a second clip over the defect.

Limitations of closure of gastrointestinal lesions with endoscopic clips

1. It is difficult to evaluate and ensure complete closure during an endoscopic session. Incomplete closure of a lesion can lead to minor leakage and clinical serositis. The use of contrast radiography imaging may be useful to confirm successful endoscopic closure.
2. Larger defects, a difficult endoscope position, a narrow or altered anatomy, and fibrosis can make endoscopic clip closure therapy difficult to achieve.
3. Early detachment of the clip could reopen the perforation with devastating consequences. In patients with acute perforation, close monitoring for 24 hours and immediate surgical intervention should be undertaken if patient experiences clinical deterioration.
4. Small and minor leaks owing to incomplete closure may lead to delayed complications such as abscess formation.
5. Chronic leaks and fistulae with fibrotic and inflamed edges are the main causes of a failed closure with over the scope clips.
6. Multiple clips may interfere with laparoscopic closure of a perforation.[3]
7. Mucosal lacerations and even perforations have been reported after deployment of the over the scope clips through the upper esophageal sphincter and esophagus.[11]

Therefore, care should be taken when advancing the over the scope-clips system through the upper esophageal sphincter and narrowed lumen like in the duodenum. The endoscopist should stop advancing the system if any resistance is noted during insertion.[12]

8. Device malfunction resulting in accidental release of the clip into normal issue, including the tongue,[13] or a partially released device with the clip stuck to the applicator cap have been reported.[14]

9. Removal of an over the scope clips can be challenging in case of unsuccessful closure. Argon plasma coagulation, bipolar cutting devices or direct current clip cutter are used to fracture the clip.[15,16]

Endoscopic Suturing

Endoscopic suturing has dramatically evolved over the last decade. It is a minimally invasive technique that has been approved by the US Food and Drug Administration for tissue apposition since 2011. The OverStitch endoscopic suturing system (Apollo EndoSurgery, Inc, Austin, TX) is a single-use suturing devices mounted onto a double-channel endoscope tip (GIF-2TH 180 or 160 Olympus, Inc) to allow the placement of either running or interrupted sutures under direct visualization using either permanent (polypropylene) or absorbable suture material as required, without removing the endoscope from the patient. Recently, the new OverStitch SX endoscopic suture system was introduced and is compatible with single channel flexible endoscopes.

Endoscopic suturing provides the ability to close larger defect. Sutures come in absorbable (2-0 and 3-0 polydioxanone) and nonabsorbable (2-0 and 3-0 polypropylene) types. The tissue must be healthy and strong to hold the sutures when they are cinched.

Characteristics of the OverStitch system

The OverStitch system includes 3 components: the endcap; the needle driver handle, which is connected to the handle control that is attached to the double working channel; and the anchor exchange catheter (**Fig. 4**). The endcap has a curved hollow needle body that opens and closes in an arc-like manner. The needle design is curved to control the depth of the suture placement and to allow for full-thickness suturing. The needle body is controlled by the needle driver handle, which is squeezed to actuate the needle driver. The anchor suture acts as the tip of the suture needle to drive the suture material through the edge of the defect for suturing.

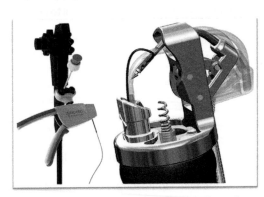

Fig. 4. OverStitch endoscopic suturing system. (*Courtesy* Apollo Endosurgery, Inc., Austin TX; with permission.)

Assist Devices

There are 3 instruments that are needed to perform endoscopic suturing: a suture cassette, a cinch device, and a helix. The tissue helix is used to acquire tissue by rotating the device handle into the target tissue until tissue is gathered into the exposed helix coil. The cinch device has thermoplastic, stainless steel materials and implantable PEEK designed to secure the placed suture.

The OverStitch technique

The endcap is attached to the distal tip of the double therapeutic endoscope. The needle driver handle is attached to the working channel. The endoscope with the closed suturing arm are advanced to the site of interest.

To load the needle body, close the needle driver handle and advance the anchor exchange catheter until the anchor clicks onto the needle body. Press the blue button and pull back the anchor exchange catheter approximately 1 cm to disengage the anchor from the anchor exchange catheter, then open the needle driver handle.

For full-thickness suturing, a tissue helix is advanced through the second working channel to the edge of the defect. Push down on the blue cross button on the helix catheter to expose the helix coil, using a forward pressure turn the helix knob clockwise to grasp the tissue. To ensure full-thickness bite, manipulate the endoscope shaft to move the tissue across the needle guard. Then retract the tissue to the endoscope tip, close the tissue handle driver to advance the anchor, and the suture through the tissue. Next, advance the anchor exchange catheter over the anchor until the locking mechanism is engaged. Once the suture is deployed through tissue, pull back the anchor exchange without pressing the blue button to disengage the anchor from the needle body. Ask your assistant to turn the helix catheter counterclockwise to release it from the tissue and pull the blue button on the helix to retract it. Finally, open the needle driver handle. Repeat the steps for additional suture bites.[17] To prepare for cinching, advance the anchor exchange catheter approximately 3 cm beyond the endcap. Press the blue button to release the anchor (T-tag). Then remove the anchor exchange catheter while keeping the suture in place. The assistant thread approximately 3 cm of the distal end of the suture through the gold suture loading loop then pull the gold tap carefully until the suture passes through the PEEK collar. Pass the cinch catheter into the working channel while your assistant holding the suture with slight tension. Advanced the cinch catheter approximately 3 cm beyond the scope tip into the first bite. To tighten the suture, apply tension to the suture with small increasing increment of force while holding the cinch catheter in place. Care should be taken not to pull the suture too tight, which may result in suture breaking. Once the desired amount of tension is reached, ask your assistant to open the cinch handle with the palm facing down to release the safety mechanism. Squeeze the cinch handle with 1 hand to pull the PEEK into the collar and lock the suture, then further squeeze with 2 hand to activate the suture cutter and release the cinch (**Fig. 5**).

Advantages of endoscopic suturing

1. Ability to perform full-thickness stitches without withdrawing the endoscope from the patient.
2. The suturing is completed with the equivalence to intracorporeal knot tying, using a cinching device.
3. Ability to close larger and chronic defects.

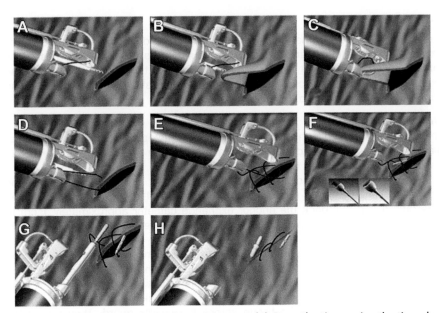

Fig. 5. Steps involved in placing endoscopic sutures. (*A*) Grasp the tissue using the tissue helix. (*B*) Retract the tissue into the needle path. (*C*) Drive the needle through the tissue. (*D*) Open the arm and release the tissue. (*E*) Repeat stitches as desired. (*F*) Press the blue button to release the needle (T-tag). (*G*) Tighten and cinch. (*H*) Repeat as desired. (*Courtesy of Apollo Endosurgery, Inc, Austin TX; with permission.*)

Limitation of endoscopic suturing

Endoscopic suturing is a more complex technique than application of clipping devices and requires advanced additional training and considerable expertise on the part of the endoscopist.

Simulators for endoscopic clipping and suturing

Limited data exist regarding the learning curves for both endoscopic clip application and suturing for closure of GI defects. For clipping, a study by Jensen and colleagues[18] found that there was a short learning curve for clip application, with trainees deploying approximately 8 hemoclips (tested for Resolution Clip, TriClip, QuickClip2) for practice before successfully assuring endoscopic placement. In a single endoscopist study evaluating the efficiency of endoscopic sleeve gastroplasty, Saumoy and colleagues[19] found that an experienced endoscopist with no prior experience in endoscopic suturing reached procedural efficiency, which was defined as the point on the learning curve where the operator was able to make procedural improvements to decrease procedure time, after 29 to 38 procedures. Further studies are needed to establish the learning curves for both suturing and clipping for the endoscopic closure of GI defects.

Additionally, endoscopic clipping and suturing can be learned through the use of synthetic simulators and ex vivo porcine organs. Simulators have been proven to be effective for training endoscopic techniques ranging from basic scope handling to advanced therapeutic interventions, such as endoscopic submucosal dissection and endoscopic mucosal resection. Maiss and colleagues[20] have successfully shown the feasibility of simulator training in teaching novices hemostatic clipping for ulcer bleeding, improving their average scores and application times significantly within a 1-month training period. Similarly for suturing, Skinner and colleagues[21] have developed and validated a synthetic and reusable simulator to learn suturing patterns used in endoscopic gastric outlet reduction after a Roux-en-Y gastric bypass. However, there remains a current lack of validated simulators for learning endoscopic clipping and suturing for the closure of GI defects. Without the widespread availability of such simulators, endoscopists are encouraged to use video-based instructional resources online and attend live workshops.[22,23]

POSTENDOSCOPIC CLOSURE CARE

Thorough inspection of the closure site after endoscopic closure is essential to ensure complete and adequate closure of the defect. Close collaboration with the surgical team is required in patients with GI defects. After successful endoscopic closure, patients need to be observed for any signs of serositis. It is critical to involve the surgeon right from the beginning as early surgical intervention, when needed, is paramount for optimal patient outcomes. Immediate surgical intervention should be undertaken if there is deterioration within 24 hours or in patients with persistent leakage after contrast imaging. Patients are typically kept nil per os initially and broad-spectrum antibiotics are administered. Nasogastric tube placement with intermittent suction of luminal secretion keeps the gut lumen collapsed and prevent leakage of GI juices through any smaller defect after clips closure. Total parenteral nutrition may be considered in patients with large defects. Contrast radiologic imaging to confirm closure is essential before resuming oral intake.

SUMMARY

Endoscopic closure of GI defects is widely practiced and is a minimally invasive alternative to the surgical approach. Extensive knowledge about medical, endoscopic and surgical principles of managing these patients is crucial. Specifically, endoscopic closure requires familiarity with various closure devices and techniques. The endoscopist should gain expertise with the variety of available closure equipment as treatment needs to be individualized and multiple techniques and accessories may be needed for management of challenging defects. TTSCs are typically used for closure of small acute perforations. Larger perforations and chronic defects (leaks and fistulae) require more advanced closure devices, such as over the scope clips, suturing, and/or stenting.

REFERENCES

1. Kumar N, Thompson CC. Endoscopic therapy for postoperative leaks and fistulae. Gastrointest Endosc Clin N Am 2013;23:123–36.
2. Magdeburg R, Collet P, Post S, et al. Endoclipping of iatrogenic colonic perforation to avoid surgery. Surg Endosc 2008;22:1500–4.
3. Cho SB, Lee WS, Joo YE, et al. Therapeutic options for iatrogenic colon perforation: feasibility of endoscopic clip closure and predictors of the need for early surgery. Surg Endosc 2012;26:473–9.
4. Willingham FF, Buscaglia JM. Endoscopic management of gastrointestinal leaks and fistulae. Clin Gastroenterol Hepatol 2015;13:1714–21.
5. Raju GS. Endoscopic clip closure of gastrointestinal perforations, fistulae, and leaks. Dig Endosc 2014;26(Suppl 1):95–104.

6. Rustagi T, McCarty TR, Aslanian HR. Endoscopic treatment of gastrointestinal perforations, leaks, and fistulae. J Clin Gastroenterol 2015;49:804–9.

7. Matthes K, Jung Y, Kato M, et al. Efficacy of full-thickness GI perforation closure with a novel over-the-scope clip application device: an animal study. Gastrointest Endosc 2011;74:1369–75.

8. Kirschniak A, Kratt T, Stuker D, et al. A new endoscopic over-the-scope clip system for treatment of lesions and bleeding in the GI tract: first clinical experiences. Gastrointest Endosc 2007;66:162–7.

9. Sandmann M, Heike M, Faehndrich M. Application of the OTSC system for the closure of fistulas, anastomosal leakages and perforations within the gastrointestinal tract. Z Gastroenterol 2011;49:981–5.

10. Albert JG, Friedrich-Rust M, Woeste G, et al. Benefit of a clipping device in use in intestinal bleeding and intestinal leakage. Gastrointest Endosc 2011;74:389–97.

11. Seebach L, Bauerfeind P, Gubler C. "Sparing the surgeon": clinical experience with over-the-scope clips for gastrointestinal perforation. Endoscopy 2010;42:1108–11.

12. Voermans RP, Le Moine O, von Renteln D, et al. Efficacy of endoscopic closure of acute perforations of the gastrointestinal tract. Clin Gastroenterol Hepatol 2012;10:603–8.

13. Honegger C, Valli PV, Wiegand N, et al. Establishment of Over-The-Scope-Clips (OTSC(R)) in daily endoscopic routine. United Eur Gastroenterol J 2017;5:247–54.

14. von Renteln D, Denzer UW, Schachschal G, et al. Endoscopic closure of GI fistulae by using an over-the-scope clip (with videos). Gastrointest Endosc 2010;72:1289–96.

15. Bauder M, Meier B, Caca K, et al. Endoscopic removal of over-the-scope clips: clinical experience with a bipolar cutting device. United Eur Gastroenterol J 2017;5:479–84.

16. Kapadia S, Nagula S, Kumta NA. Argon plasma coagulation for successful fragmentation and removal of an over-the-scope clip. Dig Endosc 2017;29:820–1.

17. Committee AT, Banerjee S, Barth BA, et al. Endoscopic closure devices. Gastrointest Endosc 2012;76:244–51.

18. Jensen DM, Machicado GA, Hirabayashi K. Randomized controlled study of 3 different types of hemoclips for hemostasis of bleeding canine acute gastric ulcers. Gastrointest Endosc 2006;64:768–73.

19. Saumoy M, Schneider Y, Zhou XK, et al. A single-operator learning curse analysis for the endoscopic sleeve gastroplasty. Gastrointest Endosc 2018;87:442–7.

20. Maiss J, Millermann L, Heinemann K, et al. The compactEASIE is a feasible training model for endoscopic novices: a prospective randomised trial. Dig Liver Dis 2007;39:70–8 [discussion: 79–80].

21. Skinner MJ, Aihara H, Jirapinyo P, et al. Development and initial validation of a fully synthetic and reusable endoscopic suturing simulator. Gastrointest Endosc 2017;85(5):AB502–3.

22. Raju GS, Saito Y, Matsuda T, et al. Endoscopic management of colonoscopic perforations(with videos). Gastrointest Endosc 2011;74:1380–8.

23. Han S, Wani S, Kaltenbach T, et al. Endoscopic suturing for closure of endoscopic submucosal dissection defects. VideoGIE 2019;4:310–3.

Printed and bound by CPI Group (UK) Ltd, Croydon, CR0 4YY

08/05/2025

01864691-0002